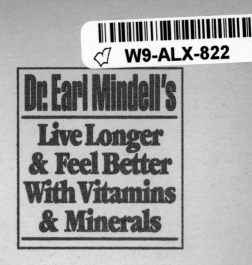

Dr. Earl Mindell's

Live Longer & Feel Better With Vitamins & Minerals

Keats Titles of Related Interest

Dr. Earl Mindell's

Live Longer & Feel Better With Vitamins & Minerals

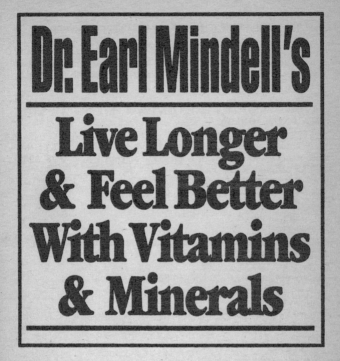

Keats Publishing, Inc. New Canaan, Connecticut

DR. EARL MINDELL'S LIVE LONGER & FEEL BETTER WITH VITAMINS & MINERALS

This book is a substantially revised and enlarged edition of the author's *Quick & Easy Guide to Better Health*, copyright © 1978, 1982 by Earl Mindell, R.Ph., Ph.D.

Library of Congress Cataloging-in-Publication Data

Mindell, Earl.
  [Live longer & feel better with vitamins & minerals]
  Dr. Earl Mindell's live longer & feel better with vitamins & minerals.
    p. cm.
  Includes index.
  ISBN: 0-87983-652-0 : $4.95
  1. Vitamins in human nutrition—Popular works. 2. Minerals in human nutrition—Popular works. I. Title. II. Title: Doctor Earl Mindell's live longer & feel better with vitamins & minerals. III. Title. Live longer and feel better with vitamins & minerals.
RA784.M513 1994
613.2—dc20   94-12737
                                                                  CIP

Printed in the United States of America

Published by Keats Publishing, Inc.
27 Pine Street (Box 876)
New Canaan, Connecticut 06840-0876

Contents

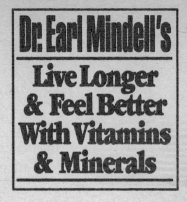

Dr. Earl Mindell's
Live Longer & Feel Better With Vitamins & Minerals

Supplements—
Why, When, How and Which

Why Take Vitamins?

It is of the utmost importance for you to understand the nutritional role that vitamins play in sustaining our bodies and our quality of life. If you were to ask a random sampling of people why they take vitamins, you would probably hear something like this:

"I take vitamins because I need them."
"I take vitamins because everyone I know takes them."
"If there's something in it for me, I want it."
"I take vitamins because my wife makes me."
"My doctor told me to take them."
"I had an ailment and found improvement after taking vitamins."
"I read a book on nutrition that recommended taking vitamins."
"I saw a doctor on television who advocated them."

Vitamins occur in all organic material. Some organic matter contains more of one vitamin than another, and in greater or lesser amounts. Therefore you might say, if I eat the "right" foods or a well-balanced diet, I will get all the vitamins I need. You are right. However, very few of us do eat this mythical diet.

First of all, much of the soil our food is grown in has been depleted of many vitamins and minerals, thanks to the overuse of fertilizers and chemicals. Then the food takes a long time to get to the supermarket—it may be stored for weeks or months before it reaches your shopping cart. The longer these foods are stored, the more vitamins they lose. Many of the foods we eat have been heavily processed, meaning they have been crushed, heated, bleached, extracted, chemicalized and preserved. Examples are most frozen foods, luncheon meats, chips, baked goods such as cookies, pies and cakes, white bread, many cereals, and some cheeses [Velveeta, for example]. Then we cook the food, destroying valuable enzymes and what's left of many vitamins. It's a wonder there's any nutrition at all left in our food by the time it gets to our tables! The term "enriched" is seen everywhere. This means that almost all the vitamins and minerals have been extracted and a few synthetic nutrients have been added to keep the government happy.

A recent University of California at Berkeley study of nearly 6,000 people in the United States showed that 70 percent of men and 80 percent of women were eating foods that contained less than two-thirds of the Recommended Dietary Allowance (RDA) of one or more of the 15 vitamins and minerals considered essential to health. One researcher added that when excess fat is added to these inadequate diets, 98 percent of these people are undernourished. The vitamins in shortest supply were A, E, C, B6 and folic acid, along with the minerals calcium, zinc and magnesium.

When and How to Take Vitamins

Since vitamins are foods—hence the term "food supplement"—they are best absorbed when taken with others foods and minerals. The human body operates on a twenty-four hour cycle. Your cells do not go to sleep when you do, nor can they exist without continuous oxygen and nutrients. Therefore, for best results with vitamins, space them out as evenly as possible during the day. The best time to take supplements is after meals, and as evenly throughout the day as possible.

Since the water-soluble vitamins, especially the B complex and C, can be excreted in the urine, a regimen taking your vitamins after breakfast, after lunch and after dinner will give you the highest body level of nutrients. If you must take your vitamins all at one time, taking them after the largest meal of the day will usually give the best results.

Minerals and vitamins are mutually dependent upon each other for proper absorption. For example, vitamin C aids in the absorption of iron. Calcium aids in the absorption of vitamin D, and zinc aids in the absorption of vitamin A. So take your minerals and vitamins together.

How Long Do Vitamins Last?

Vitamins should be stored in a cool, dark place away from direct sunlight, in a well-closed container. They do not have to be stored in the refrigerator unless you live in a very warm climate without air conditioning.

Vitamins should be guarded from excessive moisture. When you open your container, place a few kernels of rice at the bottom of the bottle. Rice works as a natural absorber of moisture.

If vitamins are kept cool and away from light in a well-sealed container, they should last for two to three years. Once a bottle is opened, you can expect twelve months of shelf life.

Today all labels should have an expiration date and manufacture's lot number. If the bottle you are buying does not, buy another brand.

Are Timed Release Vitamins Better?

The B complex and vitamin C are water-soluble. They cannot be stored in the body as fat-soluble vitamins can. Therefore they are quickly absorbed in the bloodstream and rapidly, within two to three hours, are excreted in the urine, no matter how large the dose.

Timed release vitamins are made by a process in which vitamins are enclosed in their own micropellets or tiny time pills. They are then combined into a special base for their release in a pattern that assures absorption over six to twelve hours. This gradual absorption allows the tissues greater utilization of the vitamins. I prefer the timed release form.

Why Take Chelated Minerals? What Are They?

Chelation is the process by which mineral substances are combined with amino acids and changed into their digestible form. Common mineral supplements such as bone meal and dolomite are not chelated and must be acted upon in the digestive process to form chelates before they are useful to the body.

Chelated supplements are made by the same process nature uses to chelate minerals in the body. Many people cannot perform the chelating process efficiently in their bodies, so that many of the mineral supplements they take are of little use.

Are Minerals as Important as Vitamins?

Yes! The body can synthesize some vitamins, but it cannot manufacture a single mineral. Yet minerals are biological activators necessary to the body. For example, magnesium is involved in 78 percent of our known enzyme systems.

Vitamin Notes

Some 50 to 70 percent of Americans do not meet the U.S. RDA (Recommended Dietary Allowance) for at least one or more of these vitamins:

- ♦ A
- ♦ C
- ♦ B1 (thiamin)
- ♦ B2 (riboflavin)
- ♦ Folic acid

Dieters or meal skippers usually eliminate foods that contain many vitamins, including C, E and the B complex. Sickness, including fevers and colds, can lower the level of vitamins in your blood. Senior citizens, who have difficulty chewing and digesting their food often, have poor eating habits. This condition can lead to an insufficiency of water-soluble vitamins, including B complex and C; and long-term antibiotic users can be depleted in the B complex. Prescription drugs can deplete the body of many vitamins. I'll give you specifics on those at the end of the book.

The Vitamins and Minerals

Here is a vitamin-mineral list for quick reference to the natural sources of the vitamins and minerals: what they do in the body and their deficiency signs. The deficiency symptoms described in these pages could occur only when the daily intake of the vitamins has been less than the minimum requirements over a prolonged period. These nonspecific symptoms do not alone prove a nutritional deficiency, but may be caused by any number of conditions or have functional causes. If these symptoms persist, they may indicate a condition other than a vitamin or mineral deficiency.

VITAMIN A (Beta Carotene)

ALSO CALLED

Also known as the anti-infective vitamin because it can help fight infections, and the ophthalmic vitamin because it helps improve eyesight. Vitamin A is usually measured in U.S.P. units. Beta carotene is a precursor to vitamin A, is sometimes easier for the body to absorb, and isn't toxic at high doses, as vitamin A can be. Beta carotene is a potent antioxidant. Many recent studies have shown that people who have plenty of beta carotene in their diet have a lower rate of cancer and coronary artery disease.

How It Can Help You:

- A powerful antioxidant that can slow the aging process, and help prevent disease, especially cancer and heart disease
- Builds resistance to infections, especially of the respiratory tract
- Maintains a healthy condition of the outer layers of many tissues and organs
- Promotes growth and vitality
- Permits formation of visual purple in the eye, counteracting night blindness and weak eyesight
- Promotes healthy skin
- Essential for pregnancy and lactation
- Lowers your risk of heart disease and lung, stomach and oral cancers
- Aids in the proper function of the immune system
- Shortens the duration of disease
- Promotes strong bones, healthy hair, teeth and gums
- Helps treat acne, superficial wrinkles, impetigo, boils and open ulcers

Deficiency
May result in night blindness, increased susceptibility to infections, dry and scaly skin, lack of appetite and vigor, defective teeth and gums, retarded growth.

Natural Sources
Colored fruits and vegetables, dairy products, eggs, fish oils, liver. One carrot can deliver up to 15,000 IU

of beta carotene. Add a carrot a day to your apple a day!

HOW MUCH TO TAKE
Take 10,000–25,000 IU of beta carotene or 800 to 1,000 IU daily of vitamin A daily.

VITAMIN B1

ALSO CALLED
Thiamin, thiamin chloride. Also known as the antineuritis or anti-beriberi vitamin. Vitamin B1 is measured in milligrams (mg).

HOW IT CAN HELP YOU

- ♦ Promotes growth
- ♦ Aids digestion, especially of carbohydrates
- ♦ Can improve your mental attitude
- ♦ Can help fight sea- and airsickness
- ♦ Relieves dental postoperative pain
- ♦ Aids in the treatment of shingles
- ♦ Smokers, drinkers, heavy sugar consumers, antacid users and those on birth control pills need more B1
- ♦ Is essential for normal functioning of nerve tissues, muscles and heart
- ♦ Repels insects, especially mosquitoes

DEFICIENCY
May lead to loss of appetite, weakness and lassitude (this can include anorexia), nervous irritability, insomnia, loss of weight, vague aches and pains, mental depression and constipation. In children, deficiency may cause impaired growth.

NATURAL SOURCES
Dried yeast, rice husks, whole wheat, oatmeal, peanuts, pork, most vegetables, milk.

How Much to Take
Children should take 100 mg daily, adults 200-300 mg. B1 is best taken in combination with the other B vitamins, in a B-vitamin complex supplement.

VITAMIN B2

Also Called
Riboflavin or vitamin G. Vitamin B2 is measured in milligrams (mg).

How It Can Help You
Aids in growth and reproduction
Promotes healthy hair, skin and nails
Alleviates eye fatigue
Eliminates soreness of mouth and lips
Helps your body burn carbohydrates, fats and proteins

Deficiency
A deficiency of vitamin B2 may cause a decreased ability to generate antibodies, which help the body resist disease. A deficiency may also result in itching and burning of the eyes, cracking of the corners of the lips, inflammation of the mouth, bloodshot eyes, purplish tongue.

Natural Sources
Natural sources of vitamin B2 include liver, kidney, milk, yeast, cheese, and most B1 sources.

VITAMIN B3

Also Called
Nicotinic acid (niacin), niacinamide (nicotinamide). Vitamin B3 is measured in milligrams (mg).

What It Can Do For You

 ♦ Niacin is very effective in lowering LDL or

"bad" cholesterol and raising HDL or "good" cholesterol. (If your physician has you on cholesterol-lowering drugs, don't stop taking them without supervision.)

♦ Aids in promoting a healthy digestive system
♦ Gives you healthy skin
♦ Can prevent or ease the severity of migraine headaches
♦ Increases circulation, especially in the upper body
♦ Can reduce high blood pressure
♦ Is an antidiarrheal
♦ Increases your energy through proper food utilization
♦ Helps fight canker sores
♦ Helps fight bad breath
♦ Is a possible cancer inhibitor
♦ Necessary for the metabolism of sugar

NATURAL SOURCES
Liver, lean meat, whole wheat products, yeast, green vegetables, beans.

DEFICIENCY
May result in pellagra, with symptoms including inflammation of the skin and tongue. Deficiency symptoms may also include gastrointestinal disturbance, nervous system dysfunction, headaches, fatigue, mental depression, vague aches and pains, irritability, loss of appetite, neuritis, loss of weight, insomnia, general weakness.

AMOUNTS
The usual amount taken is 50-100 mg daily. I recommend that if you have high cholesterol you take one 400 mg capsule with meals (3 times daily). If you are under the care of a health care professional for high cholesterol, please consult with that person before taking niacin to reduce cholesterol.

Niacin is a vasodilator, meaning it expands the blood vessels, bringing more blood into the upper part of the body. In large doses it can cause a "niacin flush" around the head, neck and shoulders. The skin becomes flushed and red, and this is accompanied by a burning or tingling sensation, which most people find uncomfortable and annoying. Niacinamide is more often used than niacin since it minimizes the burning, flushing and itching of the skin that frequently occurs with nicotinic acid. More recently, some vitamin manufacturers have developed "no-flush" niacin formulas that deliver all of the benefits of niacin without the unpleasant side effects. These formulas are made by combining niacin with inositol hexanicotinate, an ester involved in sending messages within the nervous system.

VITAMIN B6

Also Called

This vitamin is actually a group of vitamins called pyridoxine, pyridoxal and pyridoxamine, but B6 is often just called pyridoxine. It is measured in milligrams (mg). If it is designated in micrograms (mcg), remember that it requires 1000 micrograms to equal 1.0 milligram.

How It Can Help You

- ♦ Helps assimilate protein and fat
- ♦ Aids in converting tryptophan to niacin
- ♦ Antinauseant, including morning sickness
- ♦ Can help with PMS symptoms
- ♦ Helps synthesize anti-aging nucleic acids
- ♦ Reduces "cotton mouth" and urination problems caused by tricyclic antidepressant drugs

- ♦ Reduces night muscle spasms, leg cramps and hand numbness
- ♦ Works as a natural diuretic

NATURAL SOURCES
Meat, fish, wheat germ, egg yolk, cantaloupe, cabbage, milk, yeast, soy products, peanuts, brown rice.

DEFICIENCY
May result in nervousness, insomnia, skin eruptions, loss of muscular control.

AMOUNT
Available in doses from 50 to 500 mg. Women taking birth control pills need 4 mg daily. If your diet is high in protein, or if you are taking prescription drugs, you also need more vitamin B6. Vitamin B6 supplements have been shown to decrease a diabetic's need for insulin, so if you are diabetic, please take this vitamin only under the supervision of a physician.

YOU SHOULD KNOW
Vitamin B6 can be toxic in high doses. Please don't take more than 500 mg a day.

VITAMIN B12

ALSO CALLED
Commonly known as the "red vitamin," cobalamin. Since it is so effective in small doses, it is one of the few vitamins generally expressed in micrograms (mcg).

HOW IT CAN HELP YOU

- ♦ Forms and regenerates red blood cells which carry oxygen to the tissues, giving you more energy and preventing anemia
- ♦ Promotes growth and gives children an increased appetite

- Important for maintenance of a healthy nervous system
- Relieves irritability
- Improves circulation, memory and balance
- Can enhance immunity in the elderly, may help prevent neural tubular defects (spina bifida) in the fetus

NATURAL SOURCES
Liver, beef, pork, eggs, milk, cheese.

DEFICIENCY
May lead to nutritional and pernicious anemia, tiredness, poor appetite and growth failure in children. Women taking birth control pills need 4 mcg daily.

AMOUNT
The recommended adult dose is 2 mcg. Pregnant women should take 2.2 mcg, and nursing mothers should take 2.6 mcg. Vitamin B12 is now available as a nasal gel that seems to be absorbed better than orally taken forms.

YOU SHOULD KNOW
Vitamin B12 is only found in animal foods in any significant amounts, so if you are a vegetarian, it is important to take a supplement containing B12. Like most of the B vitamins, B12 is not well absorbed on its own, and needs to be combined with calcium in the body to be absorbed properly.

VITAMIN B15

ALSO CALLED
Pangamic acid. This controversial member of the B-complex family is highly regarded in Russia.

How It Can Help You

♦ Extends cell life span
♦ Neutralizes the craving for alcohol
♦ Speeds recovery from fatigue
♦ Lowers blood serum cholesterol
♦ Aids protein synthesis
♦ Works as an antioxidant

Natural Sources

Liver, apricot kernels, rice bran, seeds, brewer's yeast.

Deficiency

Symptoms are not known.

Amount

Vitamin B15 is most often taken in doses of 50-150 mg.

BIOTIN

Also Called

Coenzyme R or vitamin H. This one of the more recently discovered members of the B-complex family. It is measured in micrograms (mcg).

How It Can Help You

♦ Keeps hair from turning gray
♦ Prevents baldness
♦ Eases muscles pains
♦ Important for healthy skin

Natural Sources

Whole-grain foods, milk, yeast, vegetables, nuts. Present in minute quantities in every living cell, also synthesized by intestinal bacteria.

Deficiency

A deficiency of biotin may lead to hair loss, extreme exhaustion, drowsiness, muscle pains and loss of appetite; also a type of anemia complicated by a skin disease. Raw egg whites can prevent its absorption by the body.

Biotin is most often taken in doses 300 of mcg daily.

CHOLINE

ALSO CALLED
Lecithin, phosphatidylcholine.
Choline is actually an ingredient in lecithin. Choline is measured in milligrams (mg).

HOW IT CAN HELP YOU

- ◆ Lowers cholesterol
- ◆ Helps in transferring nerve impulses to the brain
- ◆ Helps against memory loss and "senile dementia"
- ◆ Aids the liver in removing poisons and drugs from the bloodstream
- ◆ Relaxant
- ◆ Regulates function of liver
- ◆ Necessary for normal fat metabolism
- ◆ Minimizes excessive deposits of fat in liver

NATURAL SOURCES
Egg yolks, brain, heart, green leafy vegetables and legumes, yeast, liver and wheat germ.

DEFICIENCY
May result in cirrhosis and fatty degeneration of liver, hardening of the arteries.

AMOUNT
The usual dose of choline is 500 to 1,000 mg daily.

FOLIC ACID

ALSO CALLED
One of the folates. Measured in micrograms (mcg).

HOW IT CAN HELP YOU

- Improves lactation
- Important for healthy skin
- Prevents neural tube birth defects such as spina bifida
- Can act as a pain reliever
- Delays gray hair, along with PABA and pantothenic acid
- Prevents canker sores
- Helps against anemia, along with iron, copper and vitamin C
- Essential to the formation of red blood cells by its action on the bone marrow
- Aids in protein metabolism
- Contributes to normal growth

NATURAL SOURCES
Deep green leafy vegetables, liver, kidney, yeast.

DEFICIENCY
Nutritional macrocytic anemia. In recognition of the fact that a folic acid deficiency can cause neural tube birth defects, the FDA is recommending that all women of childbearing years take 400 mcg of folic acid daily.

YOU SHOULD KNOW
If you are an alcoholic, pregnant, a senior citizen, on a low-calorie diet or have sickle cell anemia, you are more likely to be deficient in folic acid.

INOSITOL

ALSO CALLED
Myo-inositol is the nutritionally active form of inositol,

which is part of a substance called phosphatidylinositol. Measured in milligrams (mg).

How It Can Help You

- ♦ Lowers cholesterol
- ♦ Important for healthy hair; helps prevent premature falling-out of hair
- ♦ Prevents eczema
- ♦ Helps redistribute body fat
- ♦ Relaxant
- ♦ May relieve diabetic peripheral neuropathy

Natural Sources
Fruits, nuts, whole grains, milk, meat, yeast. Cantaloupe and citrus fruits are especially good sources.

Deficiency
Similar to that of choline.

Amount
The usual dose is 250-500 mg. Inositol is also found in small amounts in lecithin.

PABA

Also Called
Para-aminobenzoic acid. Belongs to the B-complex group. Measured in milligrams (mg).

How It Can Help You

- ♦ Sunburn protectant

Natural Sources
Yeast, liver, kidney, brown rice, bran, whole grains, wheat germ.

Deficiency
May cause extreme fatigue, eczema, anemia.

I do not recommend taking it as a vitamin unless it is included in doses under 30 mg in a multivitamin supplement.

What You Should Know
PABA causes an allergic reaction in some people who use sunblock lotion containing it. Taken by mouth, it can cause nausea and diarrhea in some people.

PANTOTHENIC ACID

Also Called
Panthenol, vitamin B5. A member of the B-complex family. Measured in milligrams (mg).

How It Can Help You

♦ Helps in the building of body cells
♦ Helps maintain normal skin, growth, and development of central nervous system
♦ Required for synthesis of antibodies
♦ Necessary for normal digestive processes
♦ Helps heal wounds
♦ Prevents fatigue
♦ Combats allergy and stress
♦ Fights infections by building antibodies
♦ Boosts athletic ability
♦ May help relieve arthritis symptoms

Natural Sources
Liver, kidney, yeast, eggs, wheat, bran, peas, crude molasses, whole grain cereal.

Deficiency
May lead to skin abnormalities, retarded growth, painful and burning feet, dizzy spells, digestive disturbances.

The usual dose is 300–1000 mg daily.

VITAMIN C

ALSO CALLED
Ascorbic acid. Expressed in milligrams (mg), occasionally in units. One mg equals 20 units.

HOW IT CAN HELP YOU

- A powerful antioxidant that slows the aging process and helps prevent heart disease and cancer
- Helps heal wounds
- Prevents fatigue
- Combats allergy and stress
- Fights infections by building antibodies
- Important for bleeding gums
- Lowers blood serum cholesterol
- Anticancer agent
- Prevents the production of nitrosamines (cancer-causing agents)
- Natural laxative
- Lowers the incidence of blood clots in the veins, therefore decreasing the risk of heart attack
- Decreases the severity and length of duration of the common cold
- Increases the absorption of iron
- Antiallergy effect by lowering histamine in the bloodstream
- Assists many minerals and other nutrients in entering cells
- Necessary for healthy teeth, gums and bones
- Strengthens all connective tissue
- Promotes capillary integrity

NATURAL SOURCES
Some vitamin C is found in nearly all fresh foods and meat. The following foods are especially high in vitamin C: citrus fruits, berries, greens, cabbages and peppers.

DEFICIENCY
May lead to soft gums, tooth decay, loss of appetite, muscular weakness, skin hemorrhages, capillary weakness, anemia.

AMOUNT
At least 500 mg daily. If you have allergies, chronic disease, stress, wounds, heart disease or gums that bleed easily, take at least 1,000 mg with every meal.

WHAT YOU SHOULD KNOW
Vitamin C can cause mild diarrhea in large doses. If this happens, either buy an esterified form of vitamin C, or back off the dose until the diarrhea stops. Vitamin C is easily destroyed by cooking.

VITAMIN D

ALSO CALLED
Calciferol, viosterol, ergosterol, "sunshine vitamin." Measured in U.S.P. units, IU.

HOW IT CAN HELP YOU

- Regulates the use of calcium and phosphorus in the body and is therefore necessary for the proper formation of teeth and bones; very important in infancy and childhood
- Taken with A and C, can help to prevent colds
- Used to treat conjunctivitis

NATURAL SOURCES
Fish oil, fat, dairy products, sunshine. Your body can manufacture vitamin D from the cholesterol in your

bloodstream, along with sunshine; most people are not very much in the sun, and may need a supplement.

DEFICIENCY
May lead to rickets, tooth decay, retarded growth, lack of vigor, muscular weakness.

AMOUNT
Most often taken in doses of 400 to 1,000 IU daily.

VITAMIN E

ALSO CALLED
Tocopherol. Available in several different forms. Formerly measured by weight (mg); now generally designated according to its biological activity in International Units (IU).

HOW IT CAN HELP YOU

- A powerful antioxidant; slows the aging process and helps prevent heart disease and cancer
- Promotes endurance
- Along with beta carotene, protects the lungs from pollution
- Prevents and dissolves blood clots
- Antifatigue vitamin
- Prevents scarring when used externally on the skin
- Accelerates burn healing
- Can lower blood pressure by its diuretic action
- Prevents night cramps, lazy leg and leg cramps
- Helps prevent cataracts
- Enhances the immune system
- Associated with sexual function; "tocopherol" relates to childbearing

NATURAL SOURCES
Wheat germ oil, whole grains, green leafy vegetables, vegetable oils, meat, eggs, avocados.

DEFICIENCY
May lead to increased fragility of red blood cells. In experimental animals, deficiencies led to loss of reproductive powers and muscular disorders.

AMOUNT
Today many cardiologists recommend that 400 IU of vitamin E be taken twice daily. The dry, water-dispersible (succinate) form of vitamin E is preferred for people over 40. If you have any of the symptoms described above, try taking 400 IU with every meal.

VITAMIN K

ALSO CALLED
Menadione, phylloquinone, phytonadione, menaquinone. Vitamin K is measured in micrograms (mcg).

HOW IT CAN HELP YOU

- ♦ Essential for the production of prothrombin (a substance which aids the blood in clotting); can prevent internal bleeding and hemorrhages; used before surgery
- ♦ Important to liver function
- ♦ Aids in reducing excessive menstrual flow
- ♦ May inhibit some cancer tumors
- ♦ May help protect against osteoporosis

NATURAL SOURCES
Although vitamin K is available in many fresh foods, the best sources are dairy products and vegetables. Alfalfa, soybean oil, egg yolks, yogurt and kefir are especially high in vitamin K.

Hemorrhages resulting from prolonged blood-clotting time.

AMOUNT
The usual dose would be 50 to 100 mcg daily. I recommend you don't take more than 100 mcg without the supervision of a physician.

VITAMIN P

ALSO CALLED
Citrus bioflavonoids, bioflavonoid complex, hesperidin. Measured in milligrams (mg).

HOW IT CAN HELP YOU

♦ Helps prevent bruising by strengthening capillary walls
♦ Increases the effectiveness of vitamin C by preventing it from being destroyed in the body by oxidation
♦ Beneficial in hypertension
♦ Helps build resistance in infections and colds
♦ Prevents bleeding gums

NATURAL SOURCES
Fruits, vegetables, nuts, seeds. One of the best sources is the peels and pulp of citrus fruit, especially lemon.

DEFICIENCY
Capillary fragility. Appearance of purplish spots on skin.

AMOUNT
Whatever vitamin C you are taking should be combined with a bioflavonoid complex. Each works best when combined with the other.

Getting to Know Some Important Antioxidants

WHAT IS AN ANTIOXIDANT?

The term "antioxidant" is practically a household word these days. Antioxidants are substances that help neutralize the damage of oxidation in the body. We can think of oxidation as similar to what happens to metal when it rusts, or to an apple when it turns brown. Unstable oxygen molecules go to war in the body, grabbing onto other cells in their attempt to become stable. In the process they damage cells, including the genetic coding, or DNA, in the cells. Once the process of oxidation begins, it can be hard to stop, and the consequences can range from heart disease and high blood pressure to arthritis and birth defects.

What causes oxidation? Probably dozens of things, but the biggest culprits we know of are pollutants, toxins, cigarette smoke, drugs and rancid oil. Unfortunately, the processed vegetable oils (corn, safflower, sunflower, soy, etc.) so heavily promoted for good health for the past thirty years have probably been major contributors to disease in this country. They are high in omega-6 fatty acids, which are very unstable and go rancid almost instantly when they are processed. These rancid fats wreak havoc in the body, setting loose a chain reaction of oxidation. Please either use olive oil, or buy vegetable oils that have been preserved by vitamin E so they won't go rancid.

Antioxidants such as vitamin C, vitamin E and beta carotene stop this "rusting" or oxidation process. These antioxidants also help the body fight disease and the effects of aging, yet according to a study from the University of California at Berkeley, there is evidence that Americans aren't getting enough of them. The study evaluated three national surveys of more than 13,000 Americans, and found that the majority of those surveyed were getting less than the RDA for these vitamins. I recommend you take at least 1,000 mg daily of vitamin C, 10,000-25,000 IU of beta carotene, a precursor of vitamin A, and at least 400 IU daily of vitamin E.

In a study at the University of Toronto, people with bladder cancer who took high daily doses of vitamins A (40,000 IU), B6 (100 mg), C (2000 mg) and E (400 IU) had 40 percent fewer tumors than a control group that took no vitamins, and also lived almost twice as long. Researchers concluded that high doses of vitamins may provide protection against the high recurrence rates that tend to be present with bladder cancer.

A study published in the *Journal of the American College of Nutrition* reported that a moderate dose of just 300 mg of vitamin C daily was shown to reduce the risk of developing cataracts by 33 percent. Vitamin E in 400 IU daily doses also dropped the risk.

My top four antioxidants are what I call the **ACES:** vitamins **A** (beta carotene), vitamin **C,** vitamin **E** and **S**elenium.

VITAMIN A AND BETA CAROTENE

Vitamin A is a fat-soluble vitamin measured in USP (United States Pharmacopoeia) units, IU (International Units) and RE (Retinol Equivalents). It occurs in two forms, preformed vitamin A, called retinol (found only in foods of animal origin), and provitamin A, known as carotene (provided by foods of both plant and animal origin).

Beta carotene is the preferred form of vitamin A; 10,000 to 25,000 IU daily is the usual dose. In large doses, vitamin A can be toxic because the body holds onto it, so it accumulates. However, you would have to take more than 100,000 IU daily for months to produce toxicity.

Beta Carotene

Beta carotene, a precursor to vitamin A (meaning vitamin A is formed from beta carotene), is a powerful antioxidant. Although I recommend you take a daily multivitamin that has beta carotene in it, you also get 15,000 IU of beta carotene by eating one carrot, and you get the full complement of carotenoids, the chemical family beta carotene is part of. I recommend you eat a raw carrot a day—make carrot sticks and have them for lunch, or grate the carrot into a salad. In the famous Harvard Nurses' Study, eating one carrot a day reduced the incidence of stroke by 68 percent, and the rate of lung cancer by 50 percent! Carrots also contain fiber and lower cholesterol.

Research Shows the Benefits of Vitamin A and Beta Carotene

Here are examples of just a few of the many uses of vitamin A and beta carotene:

Beta carotene can help prevent heart disease and cancer. It also prevents vitamin C from being oxidized or destroyed, so it's a good vitamin to take in combination with vitamin C. Beta carotene also has a protective effect on the mucous membranes of the mouth, nose, throat and lungs.

Vitamin A is essential to counteract night blindness and weak eyesight, and in the treatment of many eye disorders. It helps build resistance to respiratory infections and shortens the duration of diseases. This vitamin also keeps the outer layers of your tissues and organs healthy.

Beta Carotene and Cancer

In a study in the *American Journal of Clinical Nutrition,* G. A. Colditz reported that those who ate a diet high in beta carotene had a lower rate of all types of cancer.

In the *International Journal of Cancer,* C. La Vecchia reported on a study which found that dietary vitamin A was especially protective against cervical cancer.

The *New England Journal of Medicine* published a study by M. S. Menkes showing that beta carotene, vitamin A, vitamin E and selenium significantly reduced the incidence of lung cancer, even in people who smoked cigarettes.

VITAMIN C

Vitamin C is one of the most important vitamins our bodies require. Since as *homo sapiens,* our bodies don't have the ability to manufacture vitamin C, we must replace this precious vitamin every day of our lives or suffer the consequences. (Most animal life is able to synthesize its own vitamin C.)

What Is the Best Way to Take Vitamin C?

People are becoming more aware of the need to supplement their diets with extra vitamin C. Unfortunately, most people think that by taking an ordinary vitamin C tablet in the morning with their breakfast, they will be covered for the rest of the day. Actually, the vitamin C is metabolized and any excess is excreted in about two hours, depending on the quantity of food in the stomach.

It is very important to maintain a high level of vitamin C in the bloodstream, since it can be destroyed by stress, and/or any number of environmental pollutants, from cigarette smoke to carbon monoxide from exhaust fumes. You can do this by eating plenty of raw fresh fruits and vegetables (cooking destroys vitamin C), and by taking a vitamin C supplement with every meal. I actually recommend taking an antioxidant supplement that combines vitamins A, C, and E at every meal. There are a number of products on the market that combine these vitamins—ask at your local health food store or pharmacy.

If you're taking large amounts of vitamin C, you can avoid diarrhea by taking an *esterified* form of the vitamin.

How Long Will Vitamin C Last on My Shelf?

Vitamin C is very stable in tablet form. Long-term and short-term tests indicate that under normal storage conditions commercial vitamin C tablets are stable for periods in excess of five years (95 percent potency retention). But I hope your vitamin C will never be around for this long!

Do Smokers Need More Vitamin C?

Dr. Omer Pelletier, research scientist in Canada's Bureau of Nutritional Sciences, Food Directorate, Health Protection Branch in Ottawa, reported on a study done over a two-year period, involving smokers and nonsmokers of ages 20 to 64. The researchers gathered data on 812 male nonsmokers, 1,243 male smokers, 1,526 female nonsmokers, and 1,091 female smokers. The results clearly showed that cigarette smokers with dietary vitamin C intakes comparable to those of nonsmokers had lower blood serum vitamin C than nonsmokers. In another study, heavy cigarette smokers had as much as 40 percent lower blood plasma levels than nonsmokers. One cigarette destroys at least 25 mg of vitamin C. If you smoke cigarettes, and I hope you don't, I urge you to keep your intake of the ACES very high.

Vitamin C and Collagen

Vitamin C is essential for the formation of collagen in the body. Collagen is a protein substance which cements together the cells needed to make tissue.

Collagen is important to the body because:

♦ It is necessary for structural soundness of bones, teeth, connective tissue, cartilage and capillary walls
♦ It plays a role in wound and burn healing; it is necessary for the formation of healthy connective tissue used by the body to knit together a wound or burn
♦ It may play an important role in protecting the body from infection; a current theory holds that healthy collagen means stronger tissue which enables the body to resist invasion by disease microorganisms

The body's need for vitamin C appears to increase greatly during stress conditions. Emotional stress, extremely low environmental temperature, fever and infections are all stress conditions. Women taking birth control pills need an extra 1000 mg of vitamin C a day.

Vitamin C and Your Skin

After your skin is exposed to sunlight, vitamin C levels in your skin drop significantly. Cream or lotion with vitamin C in it can help you guard against skin cancer and wrinkles. Yes, you read it right, vitamin C on the skin will penetrate deeply into the skin, reducing the damage to your skin from ultraviolet light, and as a result reducing the wrinkles formed when your skin is damaged. According to a study reported in the *British Journal of Dermatology*, vitamin C applied to the skin of pigs protected them from ultraviolet light damage. By applying the vitamin C to *your* skin you get 20 times more into your skin than if you took it by mouth (but keep taking it by mouth!). Vitamin C applied this way penetrates into the skin and can't be rubbed, sweated or even washed off. The beneficial effects can last up to twenty days, but according to the pig study, the skin is most protected when the vitamin C is applied regularly.

Vitamin C and Allergies

If I could recommend only one thing to help with allergy symptoms it would be vitamin C. Dr. James A. Jackson states, ". . . vitamin C can be very effective in the treatment of many allergies. It may be used alone or with other agents." Large doses of vitamin C can decrease allergic symptoms, especially runny nose and cough.

Vitamin C performs an important antihistamine action in the body, making it a critical ally in fighting allergies. It is the body's release of histamines that causes allergic symptoms such as red, itchy eyes and sinus congestion. This essential vitamin, in which many Americans are deficient, works directly to lower histamine levels in the body and supports the immune system in many ways. During allergy season I recommend you take at least 1,000 mg of vitamin C three times daily, and if your symptoms continue or get worse, increase that to 1,000 mg every two or three hours.

Vitamin C and Asthma

According to Dr. Arend Bouhays, Yale University Lung Research Center, New Haven, Connecticut: "Oral administration of 500 mg of vitamin C reduces the airway constriction induced by inhalation of histamine in healthy adults." Vitamin C also affords protection against the airway-constrictor effects of certain textile dusts that act through release of histamine in the lungs, Dr. Bouhays adds. If histamine plays a part in promoting mucosal inflammation in acute respiratory illness, Dr. Bouhays speculates, then the antihistamine action of vitamin C might explain in part the reduced symptoms and duration of the illnesses.

Many physicians have noted that vitamin C can diminish, if not prevent completely, the symptoms of byssinosis, a lung disease which strikes textile workers who breathe fiber dust. This was proven in an actual study in which textile workers were given 250 mg of vitamin C every few hours. Those who received the vitamin C had significantly less incidence of the disease. In another study, athletes whose asthma was brought on by vigorous exercise had fewer asthma attacks when they took vitamin C just before and just after exercising.

Vitamin C and Heart Disease

Vitamin C helps reduce cholesterol levels and possibly slows arteriosclerosis. In a carefully done study, sixty geriatric patients took 1–3 grams of vitamin C daily for thirty months. During that time none had a heart attack, although each had a history of heart trouble. Of the sixty, 83 percent experienced a mild to impressive improvement in their symptoms. Other studies have shown that those who have certain types of heart disease have lower levels of vitamin C in their blood. Those who took vitamin C show a much lower risk of life-threatening blood clots.

Vitamin C and Colds and Flu

Numerous studies have shown that vitamin C gives the immune system a big boost in its job of fighting off colds and flu. Other studies show that once a cold or flu is in progress, taking vitamin C can reduce the severity of the symptoms and shorten the duration of the cold. One study discovered that patients taking 1,000 mg of vitamin C (1 gram) every day (and increasing that dose to 4 grams at the onset of a cold), had a 9 percent reduction in colds frequency and a 14 percent reduction in sick days.

In another fascinating study, it was discovered that although researchers could not prevent the incidence of colds in a Navajo Indian boarding school, they could decrease the sick days due to respiratory illness by 28–34 percent by giving students a dose of 1,000 to 2,000 mg of vitamin C every day. They also found that vitamin C decreased by 30 percent the incidence of non-cold-related illness.

Nobel Prize recipient Dr. Linus Pauling, in his famous book *Vitamin C and the Common Cold*, suggests a dosage of vitamin C for everyone between 1 gram and 2 grams (2,000 mg) daily. When a cold starts, he suggests 5 to 10 grams.

Vitamin C and Cancer

Numerous studies have shown the protective effect of vitamin C against cancer. Over and over again, in population studies, those whose diet includes significant amounts of vitamin C are shown to have a lower risk of most kinds of cancer. Other studies show that vitamin C actually blocks the formation of certain substances in the body that cause cancer. Small studies done on the ability of vitamin C to block cervical cancer show great promise, and more research is needed. Vitamin C has also been shown to reduce the ability of cancerous cells to form in the stomach.

Most of the research on vitamin C and cancer shows that vitamin C is a *preventive* more than a cure, but vitamin C can't help being of some assistance if you're fighting cancer. Some researchers, including Dr. Linus Pauling, believe that the studies on vitamin C and cancer already in progress have been flawed, and that better studies are needed.

VITAMIN E

In 1922, at the University of California, a substance was found to be an antisterility factor. Two years later, this substance was named vitamin E. Vitamin E was assigned its chemical name, tocopherol, around 1936, when it was isolated from wheat germ oil. Tocopherol comes from the Greek *toco*, meaning childbirth, and *phero*, meaning to bring forth. All research up to the present indicates that only alpha tocopherol is biologically active. Since alpha tocopherol is unstable, it is stabilized with acetic acid to produce alpha tocopherol acetate, which converts in the body to alpha tocopherol.

The Shute brothers, both physicians, recommended vitamin E in the 1970s as a prevention against heart disease, but for twenty years their findings were rejected by the medical establishment. Today we are now scientifically proving that vitamin E plays an important role in the maintenance of health, and particularly in a healthy heart.

For over 25 years I have been urging you to take a supplement of vitamin E daily. (I recommend you take vitamin E in the form of d-alpha tocopherol dry, or succinate form, 400 to 800 IU daily.) The reason I recommend the dry natural form of vitamin E is twofold. First, natural vitamin E is 36 percent more potent than its synthetic form (d-alpha is natural, d, l is the synthetic form.) Secondly, the dry form is easier to assimilate, especially for people over 40.

In the past few years, dozens of studies have been done showing that vitamin E is a powerful antioxidant that can prevent and reverse heart disease, prevent cancer and slow down the aging process by preventing oxidation (rusting) of the cells. A three-year study done in Japan with 1,160 people showed 82 percent of the subjects had recurrence of strokes if they were not taking vitamin E and nicotinate (a form of niacin). Those taking the tocopherol nicotinate only had a 5.9 percent recurrence rate.

Vitamin E can help protect the lungs and other air passageways against environmental pollutants such as air pollution, pesticides, and industrial pollutants. It is also a powerful and fast wound healer.

A vitamin E deficiency decreases the production of all pituitary hormones; of ACTH, essential to stimulate the adrenals, and the hormones which stimulate the thyroid and sex glands.

Vitamin E and Wound Healing

Vitamin E has also been used successfully in treating burns. It accelerates the healing rate of burns and lessens the formation of scar tissue. When applied to the skin, the antioxidizing effect of vitamin E prevents bacteria from growing.

Vitamin E and Heart Disease

Dozens of studies have been done showing that vitamin E can prevent and even reverse many kinds of heart disease. A Harvard University study of 130,000 men and women found that daily doses of vitamin E of 100 IU or more taken for at least two years, resulted in a whopping 46 percent lower heart disease risk for women and a 25 percent lower risk for men. Even the medical establishment has jumped on the vitamin E bandwagon, with many M.D.s routinely prescribing it for their patients.

Here are a few of the effects vitamin E has on the cardiovascular system. It:

♦ Is a natural anticoagulant, dissolving blood clots safely
♦ Permeates the tiny capillaries, assisting in bringing nourishment to all body cells and thereby supplying oxygen to the muscles (especially the heart muscles)
♦ Prevents undesirable excessive scarring of the heart after an infarct, while it promotes a strong "patch" scar during the healing process
♦ Is a natural vasodilator, meaning it opens up the blood vessels
♦ Allows a greater flexibility in cells and muscles, preventing hardening of the arteries
♦ Is an anticlotting agent that helps prevent blood clots in arteries and veins
♦ Helps dissolve existing clots (fibrinolytic activity)
♦ Increases the blood's available oxygen (i.e., improves the transportation of oxygen by the red blood cells)
♦ Reduces the need of the heart for oxygen by making it become a more efficient pump

Vitamin E and Diabetes

Diabetics have been found to be able to reduce their insulin levels when given vitamin E. (If you are diabetic, please check with your doctor first.)

Vitamin E and Cancer

Vitamin E has been found to prevent the growth of breast tumors. In population studies, high levels of vitamin E in the diet have been linked to a decreased risk of lung cancer and stomach cancer. In one study, two groups of hamsters were exposed to a strong carcinogen. The group given vitamin E did not get cancer, and the group that did not get vitamin E all got cancer.

Vitamin E and Neurological Disease

One of the roles of vitamin E has to do with proper neurological functioning of the body. Vitamin E has been found to be deficient in people who have many neurological diseases, including Parkinson's, cystic fibrosis and epilepsy. There is some evidence that it may help alleviate or lessen the symptoms of these types of diseases in some people. Vitamin E is an oil- or fat-soluble vitamin which means it can be stored in the liver. Toxicity studies have shown that 3,200 IU of E given daily to patients with Parkinson's disease did not produce any side effects. This therapy did show a significant slowing of the progression of the condition. Some health practitioners believe that high doses of vitamin E can even prevent or reverse some neurological diseases.

SELENIUM

Selenium is a trace mineral found in very small amounts in the body. However, its role in maintaining our health is anything but small. I have been telling you folks about this mineral for 20 years. In 1957, Dr. Klaus Schwarz and Dr. C. M. Katz established that selenium is essential to life, even though it is needed in very small quantities. Finally in 1990 it became a recommended dietary allowance (RDA) mineral. This means that your body must have this mineral daily. If we need selenium in such small amounts, why do we need to add it to our diets? White bread is one reason.

Processing grain to produce white flour robs it of 75 percent of its selenium content.

Selenium and Vitamin E

Vitamin E and selenium are synergistic, meaning that together they are stronger than they are by themselves. Selenium is also an antioxidant, so it can help to slow the aging process by preventing the damaging of tissues due to oxidation (rusting). Recent studies have shown that selenium is protective against heart disease, arthritis, liver disease, emphysema and colon cancer. Other studies have shown that selenium plays an important role in cellular immunity.

Selenium and Men

If you are male, you have a greater need for this mineral. Almost half a man's body supply of selenium concentrates in the testicles and portions of the seminal ducts adjacent to the prostate gland. Selenium is lost in semen. Blood levels of both zinc and selenium are low in men who have prostate cancer. Men who live in areas where the soil is rich in selenium tend to have lower rates of prostate cancer. If you're over the age of fifty, I suggest you supplement your diet with up to 200 mcg of selenium daily. Please do not exceed this amount, as it can be toxic in high doses.

Selenium and Colon Cancer

Over the past few years a number of studies have linked low selenium levels with colon cancer, but researchers didn't know whether that was a cause or an effect of the disease. In a more recent study at the University of Arizona, it was found that people with high levels of selenium in their blood had fewer colon polyps (growths in the lining of the colon), which are often precancerous.

Onion and garlic are a rich source of selenium, which is an important part of an antioxidant enzyme called glutathione peroxidase. This enzyme may prevent damage to cells. Some studies show that it plays a role in the repair of DNA and helps activate the immune system.

What Else Does Selenium Do for You?

♦ Aids in keeping youthful elasticity in body tissues
♦ Alleviates hot flashes and other menopausal distress
♦ Helps in treatment and prevention of dandruff

The best natural sources of selenium are: garlic, chicken, whole grains, seafood, kidneys, liver, wheat germ, bran, tuna fish, onions, tomatoes and broccoli.

SELENIUM CONCENTRATION IN HUMAN BLOOD AND HUMAN CANCER DEATH RATE IN VARIOUS CITIES

City	Blood selenium concentration mcg/100ml	Cancer deaths per 100,000
Rapid City, S.D.	25.6	94.0
Cheyenne, Wyo.	23.4	104.0
Spokane, Wash.	23.0	179.0
Fargo, N.D.	21.7	142.0
Little Rock, Ark.	20.1	176.0
Phoenix, Ariz.	19.7	126.7
Meridian, Miss.	19.5	125.0
Missoula, Mont.	19.4	174.0
El Paso, Tex.	19.2	119.0
Jacksonville, Fla.	18.8	199.0
Red Bluff, Calif.	18.2	176.0
Geneva, N.Y.	18.2	172.0
Billings, Mont.	18.0	138.0
Montpelier, Vt.	18.0	164.0
Lubbock, Tex.	17.8	115.0
Lafayette, La.	17.6	145.0

City	Blood selenium concentration mcg/100ml	Cancer deaths per 100,000
Canandaigua, N.Y.	15.7	188.0
Ontario County, N.Y.	17.6	168.0
Muncie, Ind.	15.8	169.0
Lima, Ohio	15.7	188.0

It is interesting to observe that in Rapid City, South Dakota, which has the highest blood levels of selenium in any municipality in the U.S., the cancer death rate is the lowest in the country. Coincidence? Maybe!

OTHER IMPORTANT ANTIOXIDANTS

Quercetin

You should get to know this antioxidant and anticancer agent. This bioflavonoid may also have antiviral properties. University of California laboratory studies have shown it to be a suppressant of malignant cells, which prevents them from forming tumors. Red and yellow onions are the best food sources of quercetin, though most fruits and vegetables contain some. You can also get it as a supplement. The recommended dosage of quercetin is 500 mg, 1-3 times daily.

Coenzyme Q10 (Ubiquinol)

This versatile and powerful antioxidant is the superstar when it comes to fighting "bad" or LDL cholesterol. It works well in combination with vitamin E. Co-Q10, as it is called, also regulates heart function and can work powerfully to heal gum disease. Food sources are mackerel, sardines, soybeans, peanuts and walnuts. Take two 30 mg capsules daily. All Co-Q10 is not created equal—the powder inside the capsules should be dark yellow.

THE B-COMPLEX GROUP

The B-complex vitamins help release energy from food, thus increasing available body energy to help fight fatigue. Research indicates that a deficiency of B vitamins may lead to irritability, nervousness, fear and even depression. Therefore, this is a group of vitamins necessary for calm nerves and mental stability. During stress conditions (disease, anxiety, trauma, post-surgery) many doctors prescribe a "stress formula" which incorporates the B complex with vitamin C.

B-complex vitamins help form healthy red blood cells that supply oxygen to the tissue. They can be used to relieve insomnia, neuritis, anemia and high cholesterol.

The B-complex group of vitamins consists of:

- Vitamin B1 (or thiamin)
- Vitamin B2 (or riboflavin)
- Vitamin B3 (or niacin, niacinamide)
- Vitamin B6 (or pyridoxine)
- Vitamin B12 (or cyanocobalamin, cobalamin)
- Folic acid (or folacin, pteroylglutamic acid)
- D-calcium pantothenate
- Pantothenic acid (pantothenate, panthenol)
- Biotin (or D-biotin)
- Para-aminobenzoic acid (or PABA)
- Choline
- Inositol
- Vitamin B15 (or calcium pangamate or pangamic acid)

LEADING MEMBERS OF THE VITAMIN B-COMPLEX FAMILY

Choline

In 1846, N. T. Gobley discovered a substance in egg yolk which contained glycerol, fatty acids (linoleic and linolenic acids), phosphorus and nitrogen. He called it lecithin.

In 1932, Dr. C. H. Best (codiscoverer of insulin) at the University of Toronto made the discovery that choline was important to nutrition. Further research proved that choline has a definite relationship to the metabolism of fats.

In 1968, Strecker isolated a nitrogenous base from lecithin which he called choline.

Choline is required by the thymus gland; it is needed for lactation and is especially important for kidney and liver function. In some cases, choline has brought about vast improvement in cases of cirrhosis of the liver caused by alcoholism. Today, choline is being prescribed for such diverse ailments as gallbladder trouble, diabetes, muscular dystrophy, glaucoma and arteriosclerosis. The best source of choline is still lecithin.

Inositol

In 1940, D. W. Wooley isolated inositol from liver. In subsequent experiments, it was found to recover hair in mice after they had lost it on certain other diets. Other reports showed that inositol was a growth stimulative to rats, chicks and dogs. Later an important relationship was established linking inositol, human metabolism and cholesterol.

Inositol has proved valuable to man as an auxiliary to vitamin E, helping to facilitate its actions in the treatment of muscular dystrophy. Inositol is also used in therapy of other nerve and muscle disorders, such as multiple sclerosis and cerebral palsy. However, there is still much to be learned about inositol.

Vitamin B6

Vitamin B6, or pyridoxine, is becoming more and more important because a growing number of scientific-clinical documentation is showing that it is critical in the circulatory system, the functioning of the nervous and musculoskeletal systems, and the regulation of hormones in the body. Furthermore, without vitamin B6, protein cannot be utilized properly by the body, so that a high-protein diet should include additional B6. It also helps utilize fats and carbohydrates and is essential to maintain and repair body tissues.

In Dr. John M. Ellis and James Presley's book, *Vitamin B6: The Doctor's Report* (Harper & Row), eight disease conditions in which B6 therapy has been used successfully were discussed. These include tingling fingers, muscle spasms during the night, leg cramps, numbness in the hands and severe pain of the arms, shoulders and chest. Dr. Ellis states that it was discovered in hospitals and clinics that B6 relieves certain forms of neuritis in the feet, arms, legs and hands. He also showed that edema (an excessive accumulation of fluid in the tissues) can be drastically reduced by vitamin B6.

Dr. Ellis also learned that hormones require an increased amount of B6 or become toxic in the absence of it. This is especially significant for pregnant and menopausal women, as well as for millions of women taking birth control pills.

The Minerals

Vitamins cannot function without the aid of minerals. Minerals are synergistic, meaning they work better together than individually. They work in partnership with hormones, enzymes, amino acids and vitamins. They are required to build and maintain the structure of the body.

Minerals are necessary for carbohydrates, proteins and fats to be broken down in digestion, built into cells and transformed into energy. Those that are currently considered essential for human nutrition are calcium, phosphorus, iron, potassium, selenium, sodium, iodine and magnesium. Processed or refined foods (for example, white flour and white sugar) are almost devoid of all trace minerals.

MINERALS AT A GLANCE

CALCIUM: Builds and maintains bones and teeth; helps blood to clot; aids vitality and endurance; regulates heart rhythm.

BORON: Helps retard bone loss in women after

menopause and works with calcium, magnesium and vitamin D to help prevent osteoporosis (brittle bones).

CHROMIUM: Works with insulin in the metabolism of sugar and helps the body utilize protein.

COBALT: Stimulant to production of red blood cells; component of vitamin B12; necessary for normal growth and appetite.

COPPER: Necessary for absorption and utilization of iron; formation of red blood cells.

FLUORINE: May decrease incidence of dental cavities.

IODINE: Necessary for proper function of thyroid gland; essential for proper growth, energy and metabolism.

IRON: Required in manufacture of hemoglobin; helps carry oxygen in the blood.

MAGNESIUM: Necessary for calcium and vitamin C metabolism; essential for normal functioning of nervous, muscular and cardiovascular system.

MANGANESE: Activates various enzymes and other minerals; related to proper utilization of vitamins B1 and E.

MOLYBDENUM: Associated with carbohydrate metabolism.

PHOSPHORUS: Needed for normal bone and tooth structure. Interrelated with action of calcium and vitamin D.

POTASSIUM: An electrolyte that helps regulate pH balance and water in the body.

SELENIUM: Trace mineral that helps prevent cancer, stimulates the immune system, and works with vitamin E.

SODIUM: Otherwise known as salt. An important electrolyte that helps regulate pH balance and water in the body.

SULFUR: Vital to good skin, hair and nails.

VANADIUM: Possible insulin-like activity. More study is needed.

ZINC: Helps normal tissue function, protein and carbohydrate metabolism.

THE ESSENTIAL MINERALS

Calcium

Calcium is by far the most important mineral the body requires, yet calcium deficiency is more prevalent than that of any other mineral. The adult body contains three to four pounds of calcium, 99 percent of which is in bones and teeth. Since it is so concentrated in the bones and teeth, only 1 percent of our calcium circulates in body fluids and tissues. When calcium intake is inadequate, some of it is stored in the ends of the bones. Under stress situations this reserve storage is used. If the body has no reserve calcium, then it is taken from the bone structure, usually the spinal and pelvic bones.

Symptoms of calcium deficiency are stunted growth, decayed teeth, and nervousness.

Calcium is vital to the nerves of the body. Without sufficient calcium in the bloodstream, nerves cannot send messages effectively. Finger tapping, impatience and quick temper can be signs of a calcium deficiency. When your grandmother gave you a glass of milk before bedtime she was wisely giving you a dose of calcium to relax your muscles and ease you into sleep.

Calcium is needed for normal blood coagulation or clotting, to activate enzymes (digestive juices) and to regulate fluid passage throughout cellular walls. It is required for every heartbeat.

Calcium helps maintain the delicate acid-alkaline body balance.

Calcium can be assimilated only by getting plenty of phosphorus, iodine, vitamin A, vitamin B and vitamin D. Adequate hydrochloric acid in the stomach is also necessary for the absorption of calcium. Calcium and phosphorus must exist in a two-to-one ratio in the body; that is, two parts calcium and one part phosphorus. Vitamin D helps to normalize and maintain a good balance of calcium and phosphorus. A two-to-one relationship is also necessary for magnesium and calcium—two parts calcium to one part magnesium.

CALCIUM AND KIDNEY STONES

We used to be told that too much calcium would cause kidney stones, because those painful pluggers are made mostly of calcium. We now know that's wrong! In the most recent study debunking that old theory, 45,000 men between the ages of 40 and 75 were evaluated for the relationship between how much calcium they had in their diet and the formation of kidney stones. At a four-year follow-up, the 505 men who had kidney stones were the ones who had a high intake of animal protein (meat and dairy products), and reduced potassium and water intake. In fact, based on other measurements in the study, the researchers concluded that getting a lot of calcium in the diet actually *decreased* the risk of kidney stones.

CALCIUM AND OSTEOPOROSIS

From the age of nine, the diets of girls and women may lack as much as 25–30 percent of the calcium they need. The diet of many young people, particularly teens, is woefully inadequate in calcium. To add insult to injury, the phosphoric acid in sodas pulls calcium out of the body. This sets up an early prognosis for osteoporosis, or thinning of the bones, which affects millions of American women after menopause. Alcohol, caffeine, smoking and sugar can also deplete the body's calcium.

Calcium is an important factor in preventing osteoporosis—everyone should have at least 1,200 mg of easy-to-absorb calcium daily. Some good sources of calcium are snow peas, broccoli; leafy green vegetables such as spinach, kale, beet and turnip greens; almonds, figs, beans (soybeans are the best); and nonfat milk, yogurt and cottage cheese. Calcium is very important, but in older women it has been found that calcium supplements only *slow* the process of bone loss. Some studies suggest that calcium depletion is only seen in about 25 percent of women with osteoporosis. Please be sure any young girls in your family are getting plenty of calcium *now*. And not from those calcium-added sugary soft drinks please!

Research has shown a direct link between a high-protein diet and calcium loss. The high phosphorous content of meat may cause the body to lose calcium in its attempt to counteract the phosphorus. The average American gets more than enough protein, so for most of us it can only help to cut down on our meat consumption.

Calcium gluconate, citrate or lactate are easy-to-absorb forms of calcium. Please avoid calcium supplements in the form of bone meal or oyster shells, as they can have a high lead content and aren't as easy for the body to absorb. Your calcium supplement should always be combined with magnesium.

Chromium

Many studies have shown that chromium lowers cholesterol. In a recent study 34 male body builders were given a chromium-and-niacin complex or a placebo. Cholesterol levels increased in the test group (placebo) and decreased in the chromium-niacin group.

Chromium also works with the body to metabolize sugar. It can work as a deterrent to diabetes and be used to treat glucose intolerance. Much more research is needed on this mighty mineral! I recommend supplementing your diet daily with 50 to 200 *micrograms* (not milligrams!) of chromium picolinate, a form of chromium easily used by the body.

Copper

Copper works as a catalyst in the formation of red blood cells and is present in the hemoglobin molecule. It also plays a role in maintaining the skeletal system. Copper must be present before iron can be utilized and is necessary to prevent anemia. It is an important partner to vitamin C in the synthesis of collagen. You don't usually need to add copper to your diet, and an excess of it can cause hair loss, insomnia, irregular menses and depression.

Fluorine

An element, also called fluoride, that helps protect teeth from decay and may help protect against osteoporosis. Too much causes discolored teeth and continued overuse of it may lead to bone fractures. Most Americans have it added to their water and don't need more than that.

Iodine

The most important fact about iodine is that a deficiency of it can cause goiter—a swelling of the thyroid gland. Kelp is a good source of natural iodine. Seafoods are very high in iodine, and it is added to most table salt. Iodine is necessary for proper function of the thyroid gland, and for proper growth, energy and metabolism. It can help dieting by burning excess fat. Iodine promotes healthy hair, nails, skin and teeth.

You should be getting 200–600 mcg daily as part of your food or in your multivitamin.

Iron

Iron is the second most deficient mineral in the human body. It is the prime factor in anemia prevention, and a key factor in healthy blood. It is the essential ingredient in hemoglobin. Without iron, the blood could not carry oxygen to the tissues. Without oxygen, the body tissues die. Iron also plays a role in food metabolism.

Women need more iron than men because of the loss of blood during the menstrual cycle. Pregnancy and breast-feeding also increase the body's demand for iron. The pregnant woman transfers iron to the growing fetus and to the placenta. This transfer of iron is heaviest during the last three months of pregnancy.

There have been numerous studies showing that athletes doing aerobic exercise deplete their iron stores and need either supplements, a diet high in iron, or both. A study of high school cross-country runners found 45 percent of the female runners and 17 percent of the male runners had low iron levels during the competitive season. Another study of 100 female college students showed that 31 percent had iron deficiency. Young women who were limiting their calories because of concerns about gaining weight were particularly susceptible. Many people run the risk of an iron-poor diet when they restrict their food intake in an effort to lose weight. Vegetarian diets also increase the likelihood that the body's need for iron will not be met. If you are a vegetarian, please be sure your daily multivitamin contains iron.

While the best food source of iron is meat, it is still best to eat lean meat in small quantities.

The most noticeable warning sign of anemia, a sign

of iron deficiency, is fatigue. If you are getting plenty of rest, but still feel tired and lacking in energy, your body could be telling you that you are becoming anemic. The hair, skin and nails also show the effects of anemia. The skin tends to wrinkle more. Fingernails and toenails become brittle and break easily, and become tender. Hair becomes dry and lacks luster. Skin color becomes paler, even pasty and gray. The mouth and tongue begin to feel sore and tender.

Fortunately, the treatment of iron-deficiency anemia is as simple as checking with your doctor and taking iron supplements.

Copper, cobalt, manganese and vitamin C are necessary to assimilate iron. B-complex vitamins such as B1, B6, biotin, folic acid and B12 all work with iron to produce rich red blood. Since inorganic iron—ferrous sulfate—destroys vitamin E and ferrous gluconate is harder for the body to assimilate, please use organic forms of iron called ferrous citrate or ferrous peptonate. Inorganic iron may cause constipation and upset stomach.

Too much iron taken over a long period of time can be toxic, so please limit your intake to 10–30 mg daily.

Magnesium

Dr. Hans Selye of McGill University called magnesium the antistress mineral. He has saved animals under great stress by giving them protective amounts of magnesium. Without the protective mineral, those animals generally died of heart damage. In controlled studies of rats, it was found that magnesium was necessary to prevent calcium deposits, kidney stones and gallstones. Magnesium is regularly used in hospital emergency rooms for heart attack victims, to help control any damage caused by the heart attack.

Magnesium deficiency may be more common in women with osteoporosis than calcium deficiency. Although many fruits and vegetables have some magnesium in them, especially good sources of magnesium are whole grains, wheat bran, leafy green vegetables, nuts (almonds are a very rich source of magnesium and calcium), beans, bananas and apricots.

Magnesium regulates calcium uptake by cells, so take a magnesium/calcium combination for the greatest effect. Take 600 mg daily of calcium citrate, and 300 mg daily of magnesium.

Potassium

Potassium is an essential mineral, like calcium and phosphorus. It is needed in somewhat the same quantities as magnesium. There must be a proper balance between sodium, calcium and potassium.

In a nutshell, potassium:

♦ Is necessary for normal muscle tone, as well as nerve, heart and enzyme reactions
♦ Aids in clear thinking by sending oxygen to the brain
♦ Helps dispose of body wastes
♦ Assists in reducing high blood pressure
♦ Aids in allergy treatment
♦ Deficiency leads to edema and hypoglycemia (low blood sugar)
♦ Is needed in increased amounts by heavy coffee drinkers and heavy sugar eaters
♦ Is needed by dieters to keep up their energy levels

Potassium is needed in many functions, but especially for heart rhythm. Aided by sodium, it also assists the cells in the selection of food particles. Both potassium and sodium help to pull the particles out of the blood, and both minerals aid the cells in the elimination of wastes. Potassium attracts the nourishment that the cells need from the bloodstream.

Organic potassium (the gluconate, the citrate, the fumarate) is preferable to the inorganic (the sulfate or alum, the chloride, the oxide and carbonate, etc.). Natural sources of potassium are primarily green leafy vegetables. Most people do not eat enough of these. Unfortunately, they are not an adequate source for any potent supply; supplements are needed.

Ninety-eight percent of the total potassium is found inside the cells, while the remaining two percent is distributed between the bloodstream and other body fluids. Potassium depletion is common during long fasts, chronic disease characterized by weight loss, and muscle atrophy. Major surgery or other major trauma such as burns, fractures, severe muscle damage or severe diarrhea also cause potassium loss.

But the most common cause of potassium loss today is manmade. It is the use of diuretic drugs ("water pills"). They are used in the treatment of edema and hypertension (high blood pressure). The problem is so common that many physicians routinely prescribe potassium supplements for long periods of time. A special supplement is needed—if you take a diuretic, consult your doctor. Other causes of potassium loss are the use of the steroid drugs, cortisone and ACTH, and chronic stress, which causes constant release of certain hormones that deplete potassium.

The symptoms of potassium loss are fatigue, muscle weakness, paralysis and frequent urination.

Sulfur

Sulfur is a blood conditioner and cleanser. It aids the liver in absorbing the other minerals. Referred to as the beauty mineral, it has been known to make the difference between stringy or shiny hair, brittle or beautiful nails, and, coupled with vitamins A and D, to play a major part in skin texture integrity.

Vanadium

Vanadium is a mineral stored mainly in our bones and fat. Although no human deficiency of vanadium has ever been identified, in test animals a deficiency caused impaired growth of teeth, bones and cartilage, thyroid changes, decreased overall growth and fluid retention. This mineral can also be used to build up teeth, bones, cartilage and even muscle. It stimulates cell division, but also has anticarcinogenic properties.

A substance called vanadyl sulfate, which is derived from vanadium, is used to increase muscle growth and development, and appears to make muscles larger and more dense more rapidly than normally would be the case.

Zinc

Think of zinc as a traffic policeman, directing and overseeing the efficient flow of body processes, the maintenance of enzyme systems, and the integrity of our cells. It is a tiny but powerful catalyst which is absolutely essential for most integral body functions. Zinc is a trace mineral found in such small amounts in our bodies that it has been called a micronutrient. It is found in the thyroid gland, hair, finger- and toe-nails, nervous system, liver, bones, pancreas, kidneys, pituitary glands, blood and in the male reproductive fluid or semen. It is the prime element in male hormone production. Zinc is a constituent of insulin, which is necessary for the utilization of sugar. It also assists food absorption through the intestinal wall.

Zinc governs the contractility of our muscles, stabilizes blood and maintains the relationship of acidity and alkalinity in the blood and other fluids. Zinc is essential for the synthesis of protein and in the action of many enzymes. A lack of zinc can cause increased fatigue, susceptibility to infection and injury, and a slowdown in alertness and scholastic achievement.

Zinc exerts a normalizing effect upon the prostate, and a lack of the mineral can produce testicular atrophy and prostate trouble. Zinc is necessary for the proper function of the prostate gland. In men, higher concentrations of this mineral are found in the prostate than anywhere else in the body. A recent study looked at zinc supplementation in young men, and found that when plasma zinc levels were low, there was a corresponding drop in testosterone. There have been many clinical studies showing that zinc supplementation can reduce the size of the prostate gland, along with troublesome symptoms.

I recommend that all men take up to 30 to 50 mg (not more than 50) of zinc daily, and include zinc-rich foods in the diet such as oysters (well-cooked, please!), lamb chops and wheat germ. Pumpkin seeds are a good source of zinc.

Most zinc available in foods is lost in processing. For example, 80 percent of the zinc in white bread is destroyed by processing. White spots or bands on fingernails may indicate zinc deficiency.

Foods rich in zinc include brewer's yeast, bone meal, beans, pumpkin and sunflower seeds, wheat germ, fertile eggs, fish and meat. Liver is an exceptional source. Zinc supplements can be taken as lozenges, and in that form can cut down the length and severity of colds and flu, especially when combined with vitamin C.

How to Improve Your Nutrition

The success of any program of nutritional therapy is founded upon a sound daily diet. In the case of disease or deficiency conditions, this is especially important, since the body must receive substantial quantities of high-quality "building blocks" such as protein to facilitate the vitamins and minerals in their action. Eliminate food items which contribute little or nothing to nutritional or physical status. Emphasize those which are beneficial.

What to Cut Down on or Eliminate

Sugar: White, brown and products containing refined sugar. Also avoid sugar substitutes (saccharin, cyclamate). Use honey or molasses sparingly. If you crave sweets, try eating sweet fruits such as grapes or bananas.

Refined flours: White, partially refined, bleached and any products such as pastry, cookies, cakes or breads containing flours of this type.

Refined grains: Hot and cold breakfast cereals and cereal products (unless prepared from unprocessed whole grain). White rice and blanched or degermed grains.

Pasta: Macaroni, noodles, spaghetti and related items, unless made from whole wheat and/or Jerusalem artichoke.

Dairy products: Some 80 percent of American adults may be lactose intolerant, that is, unable to digest the lactose in milk and other dairy products. (The most common symptoms are gas and bloating after eating.) If you can digest lactose, please stick to nonfat dairy products. Yogurt is an exception to this. Please try to find milk that says, "hormone free," and if you can't find it in your supermarket, demand it!

Fat: This means animal fat and vegetable fats. Try to satisfy your fat cravings with the fats that are good for you: Those found in fish and olive oil are the best. Those found in red meat and unpreserved vegetable oils are the worst.

Processed meats: This includes smoked foods such as ham, meats such as hot dogs preserved with nitrates and other preservatives, and luncheon meats. Best to cut these out.

Red meat: Please limit your intake of red meat to one or two meals a week, and then eat only lean meat or cut the fat off.

Frozen dinners: Those containing preservatives, additives, and sodium more than 300 mg per serving. There are plenty of delicious "health food" frozen dinners available now. Please read labels.

Dessert: Virtually all prepared, baked, processed sugar desserts. Try fruit for dessert instead.

Beverages: Alcoholic beverages, soft drinks, coffee.

Miscellaneous: All snack foods made from unpreserved vegetable oils and/or which have a high salt content. Candy products, ice cream and related items. French fries and deep-fried foods, especially when prepared in batter.

Canned fruits and vegetables: All canned fruits and

vegetables—please eat your fruit and vegetables fresh or frozen fresh!

What to Increase or Feature

Yogurt: This is a virtual wonder food, loaded with nutrition and friendly bacteria necessary for proper digestion. I suggest you eat at least one cup a day of yogurt with live cultures.

Eggs: Eggs have gotten a bad rap over cholesterol. While they do have some, it's not as high as once thought, and much of it is "good" cholesterol. Eggs are a good source of protein and many other nutrients. Enjoy them.

Whole-grain products: Wheat germ, bran, whole-grain cereals and bread, corn and other items prepared from whole oats, rye, barley, etc. Brown rice.

Meat: Eat more chicken and turkey, less beef and pork.

Seafood: Fish is wonderful, but make sure it's caught in unpolluted waters. The oily fish such as salmon, herring and mackerel are loaded with omega-3 fatty acids, which help prevent heart disease. Please eat shellfish well-cooked to avoid bacterial contamination. Avoid seafood canned in vegetable oils.

Nuts and seeds: Nuts and seeds of all varieties are healthy in moderate amounts, provided they are unsalted, and without added oil. Especially good are toasted raw almonds, cashews, pumpkin and sunflower seeds. Try to buy organic peanuts and peanut butter as they otherwise tend to be heavily polluted with pesticides.

Vegetables: Vegetables, except those just listed under "What to Cut Down on or Eliminate," should be used regularly and in abundance. Maximum benefit is obtained from fresh or frozen rather than canned varieties. Emphasis should be placed on leafy green vegetables and the cruciferous vegetables such as broccoli and cauliflower.

Legumes: If you can digest them, beans are high in protein and carbohydrates and are loaded with nutrients. Soybeans are an especially healthy food and are found in tofu, tempeh, miso and many other products.

Fruit: Eat fruit daily. Use fruit in place of unhealthy snacks and sugary desserts.

Beverages: Fruit and vegetable juices are great, but avoid added sugar. Tea in moderation, herbal teas, decaffeinated coffee, and nonfat milk are healthy beverages. And of course, pure water.

Guidelines for Nutritional Health

- Eat food slowly, chew it well and choose smaller amounts
- Light meals with healthy snacks between meals are better than big meals
- Avoid "instant" foods and products with chemical additives, colorings or compounds
- Be careful preparing foods; use olive oil instead of butter, use vegetable oils preserved with vitamin E, and minimize consumption of fried foods
- For maximum benefit, quick-steam vegetables, or prepare in a wok
- Take medication only on the advice of a physician
- Follow a program of regular exercise
- Drink 6–8 glasses of clean water daily
- Cut down on fat consumption and increase whole grains, fruits and vegetables

Basic Meal Guidelines

Breakfast (the most important meal of the day)

- Drink at least one glass of clean water as soon as you get up

- ◆ Protein (yogurt, eggs, nonfat milk on cereal, or a protein drink, for example)
- ◆ Whole-grain bread or cereal: corn, rice, wheat, oats, etc.
- ◆ Fresh fruit
- ◆ Tea (black, green or herb), juice or nonfat milk

Midmorning Snack
One of the following:

- ◆ Fruit
- ◆ Nuts
- ◆ Low-fat, low-salt chips

Lunch

- ◆ Turkey sandwich on whole-grain bread with nonfat mayonnaise (you can skip the bread if you want to cut down on calories, but a good, dense bread has fiber and is filling—and these complex carbohydrates may help prevent snack attacks later on)
- ◆ Carrot sticks
- ◆ Fruit

Midafternoon Snack
Same as midmorning.

Dinner

- ◆ Small serving of protein (chicken, turkey, fish, beans and carbohydrate such as rice, tofu, eggs, cheese, etc. Use red meat sparingly)
- ◆ Complex carbohydrate (potato, corn, whole-grain pasta, brown rice, etc.)
- ◆ 1–2 servings of vegetables
- ◆ Fruit for dessert

Do You Eat Too Much Salt? (Sodium Chloride, NaCl)
Most people in the United States today are ingesting large amounts of salt without even knowing it. Most

of us are aware that pretzels, potato chips and French fries are salty, but few of us are aware that many other foods, such as pastries, cheeses and packaged cereals, may also contain considerable amounts of salt.

Up to 25 percent of the American public has hypertension or high blood pressure. There is no doubt in my mind that our excessive ingestion of salt is an important factor contributing to high blood pressure. *Some general rules to remember to decrease your salt intake are:*

1. Avoid the use of salt at the table, as well as baking soda, monosodium glutamate (MSG, "Ac-cent") and baking powder in food preparation.
2. Avoid laxatives or other substances containing sodium.
3. Do not drink or cook with water treated by a home water softener, as these appliances add sodium to the water.

If you were on a mild sodium-restricted diet, you would be allowed 2–3 grams of sodium per day. The average American ingests 5–15 grams (approximately half an ounce) of salt daily.

The Most Powerful Natural Food Supplements

In the preceding pages, I have written about vitamin and mineral food supplements and nutrition. Now, in alphabetical order, I would like to discuss some of the truly healthy foods that, unfortunately, most Americans do not eat. Some of them have been known since Biblical days, some were discovered just a few decades ago, some are in the news today, and some we have forgotten about, entirely.

Acidophilus/Yogurt

It's a nice feeling to see a food I have been recommending for 25 years now becoming a mainstream food in all supermarkets in the U.S. I urge that everyone eat yogurt containing "live cultures" called acidophilus at least once a day, or take acidophilus capsules.

Why should you eat yogurt?

- ♦ Yogurt contains fermented cultures containing the "good" bacteria found in your digestive system. These bacteria are essential to proper digestion, and aid the body in absorbing calcium.

♦ Yogurt can help reduce cholesterol. Many recent studies indicate that the fermented cultures in yogurt help lower cholesterol.

♦ Yogurt can help your immune system do its job. It has been a folk remedy for colds, diarrhea and fighting infections for centuries, and now scientific research is validating this. There is even some evidence that eating yogurt daily can help reduce hay fever symptoms.

♦ Yogurt can help fight cancer. Research indicates that yogurt seems to block the development of cancer tumors. There's something about those "good" bacteria that inspires the immune system to destroy tumor cells.

♦ Yogurt can reduce lactose intolerance. Lactose is milk sugar that many people (some say as much as 80 percent of the adult population) have trouble digesting. Lactose intolerance can cause chronic gas, intestinal cramps and allergy symptoms. However, lactose-intolerant people who eat yogurt daily seem to develop a much greater ability to digest lactose.

♦ Yogurt can help reduce or eliminate ulcers. About 40 years ago scientists discovered that too much of a specific bacteria in the stomach causes ulcers. Unfortunately this research was ignored until recently when it was "rediscovered." The friendly bacteria in yogurt destroys the bacteria that causes ulcers and many other digestive difficulties.

♦ Yogurt can cure bad breath, which is often caused by putrefaction in the intestines that is totally resistant to mouth wash or breath spray. This condition is usually accompanied by foul-smelling flatulence. An intensive course of acidophilus culture usually solves this problem.

♦ Yogurt can help the stomach problems caused by antibiotics. Many doctors prescribe acidophilus in conjunction with oral antibiotic treatment because antibiotics destroy the friendly bacteria, causing an overgrowth of the fungus *Monilia* (or *Candida*) *albicans*. The fungus can grow in the intestines, vagina, lungs, mouth (thrush), on the fingers, or under the finger or toenails. It usually disappears after a few days of large amounts of acidophilus culture. If you take antibiotics, please be sure to follow them up with a cup of yogurt twice daily for at least two weeks, or buy acidophilus in capsules at your local health food store. You can also buy an acidophilus milkshake-like drink called kefir at most supermarkets. It usually comes in a variety of flavors.

Alfalfa

Frank Bouer, a biologist, author of *This Business of Eating*, has called alfalfa "the great healer." He discovered that the green leaves of this legume contain eight essential enzymes. Later, Dr. C. A. Jacobson, a food scientist with the U.S. government, confirmed these findings. It also seems to contain sufficient vitamin D, lime and phosphorus to make strong bones and teeth in growing children.

Alfalfa is truly valuable for its vitamin content. It contains 8000 IU of vitamin A for every 100 grams. It is a good source of vitamin B6 and vitamin E. It is extremely rich in vitamin K, which protects against hemorrhaging, and helps the blood to clot properly. Alfalfa contains about 100 mcg of vitamin K for every 100 grams.

Alfalfa has been used by doctors in treating stomach ailments, gas pains, ulcerous conditions and poor appetite. Alfalfa has natural diuretic properties (it promotes the excretion of urine) and is a natural laxative.

Bee Pollen

Throughout the ages, man has valued and made use of bee pollen as a health food and healing agent. Pollen is mentioned in the Bible, the Koran and the Talmud. Famous and learned men of old, such as the physician Hippocrates, the naturalist Pliny, and the poet Virgil, firmly believed that bee pollen had a most important role to play in making sure of good health and protecting against the many problems associated with old age.

Bee pollen contains all of the eight essential amino acids in varying amounts that fluctuate between five and seven times the amino acid content of equal weights of traditional high-protein foods. Pollen also contains vitamins A, D, E, K, and C and bioflavonoids, as well as the complete B complex, especially pantothenic acid and niacin. This may be the reason why research has shown that pollen puts up a powerful defense against stress.

In addition to all this goodness, 27 mineral salts and bio elements have been found in bee pollen, including calcium, copper, iron, magnesium, manganese, phosphorus, potassium, silicon, sodium and sulfur.

Dr. Peter Hernuss and six colleagues at the University of Vienna's Women's Clinic conducted a study involving 25 women with inoperative uterine cancer. During the course of radiotherapy, fifteen of the women received a supplement of bee pollen, and the other ten served as a control group and were subjected to radiation alone. The pollen was administered three times daily in 20-gram doses. The women receiving the pollen supplement were able to tolerate the radiation stress much better.

Dr. Emil Chauvin announced to the French Academy of Science that results of his intensive studies using bee pollen showed that pollen produced an all-round improvement in general health and increased the red blood corpuscles and hemoglobins in anemic patients. He also found it beneficial in cases of prostate problems, constipation, flatulence and infections of the colon, especially diarrhea. Dr. Chauvin also discovered that pollen contains an antibiotic which regulates the intestines by destroying or weakening harmful bacteria and at the same time promoting the growth of friendly bacteria. Bee pollen therapy builds up strength and energy in tired bodies.

Bee pollen can be used by some allergy sufferers. If taken before the onset of the allergy season, it can prevent allergy symptoms. The bee pollen may have a "vaccinating" effect on the body. Bee pollen also contains quercetin, which inhibits the release of histamines in the bloodstream, thus preventing an allergic response to allergens.

Bee pollen should be taken fifteen to twenty minutes before a meal, preferably breakfast, when the stomach is completely empty. It may be taken by persons of all ages; in fact, the older the person the more beneficial it may be. Some people who are allergic to pollens may become allergic to bee pollen. Try a small amount first to find out.

Bran

There is a correlation between a long-term dietary intake of low-fiber refined foods such as white flour and sugar, and illnesses such as heart disease, colon cancer, appendicitis, hemorrhoids, constipation and gallstones. Cultures that eat a diet high in fiber have a low to nonexistent rate of these diseases. Many of us in Western civilization would live longer and be a great deal healthier if we ate high-fiber diets that would keep our digestive system cleaned out and tuned up.

Bran has little or no food value. We do not digest and absorb it. As it passes through our digestive tract, it accumulates liquid and swells up, providing a good amount of soft bulk that speeds bowel movements.

I recommend that you eat breads, rice, pasta and cereals made of whole grains, and add unprocessed bran to your diet. Bran comes in many breakfast cereals, or it can be mixed in to hot or cold cereal and even yogurt. Fresh fruits and vegetables also have plenty of fiber. Studies suggest that eating unprocessed bran prevents gallstones and might possibly reduce the size of existing gallstones.

Chlorophyll

Chlorophyll possesses an antibacterial action, making it a good inner and outer wound-healing agent. It acts as a direct stimulant to the growth of new tissue while simultaneously reducing the hazard of bacterial contamination, thus acting as a wound-healing agent. Chlorophyll also has antioxidant properties.

Garlic

Garlic contains potassium and phosphorus, plus a significant amount of B and C vitamins, as well as calcium and protein. It also contains a number of substances that help prevent and heal all kinds of illnesses.

Many scientific studies agree that garlic reduces high blood pressure, lowers blood cholesterol and contains a substance that thins the blood, which helps prevent the formation of blood clots.

Garlic is a potent antioxidant and has also been shown to reduce cancer rates. Even the National Cancer Institute has put garlic at the top of its "foods that can prevent cancer" list. In a study done in China of two different provinces with different diets, the one that ate a lot of garlic had a much lower rate of stomach cancer than the one that had little garlic in the diet. Animal studies done in animals with induced cancer found that those fed garlic in the diet did better.

Fresh garlic, which contains a substance called allicin, also seems to have the ability to help us fight off infections, especially viral and fungal infections.

Some studies have shown that people eating garlic find their arthritis symptoms are relieved. It is thought that garlic may have an inhibitory effect on substances in the body that promote the joint inflammation of arthritis.

Garlic is a time-honored folk remedy for clearing up intestinal parasites. An Egyptian study found that children given fresh garlic or garlic capsules daily cleared up parasite symptoms in a matter of days. (Because of the cyclical nature of parasites, you would need to take garlic for a few months to completely clear out parasites.)

Kelp

Kelp, a seaweed, contains twenty-three minerals and elements:

Iodine	0.15-0.20%	Magnesium	0.76%
Calcium	1.20	Sulfur	0.93
Phosphorus	0.30	Chlorine	12.21
Iron	0.10	Copper	0.0008
Sodium	3.14	Zinc	0.0003
Potassium	0.63	Magnesium	0.0008

Vitamins present in kelp are vitamin B2, niacin, choline and carotene. Algenic acid is also present. This remarkable food contains more vitamins and minerals than any other substance. All these nutrients have been assimilated by the growing kelp plant.

Homeopathic physicians use kelp for obesity, goiter, poor digestion, flatulence and obstinate constipation.

Because of its natural iodine content, kelp acts on the thyroid gland to normalize it. Therefore, thin people with thyroid trouble may gain weight by using kelp, and obese people with thyroid trouble may lose weight.

To show you how important the thyroid gland is to human metabolism, here is a list of the thyroid functions:

♦ Secretes thyroxine
♦ Controls and regulates metabolism
♦ Vitalizes every cell of the body and enables them to respond to sympathetic stimulation
♦ Assists in control of tissue differentiation
♦ Increases the power and rate of heart function
♦ Controls coagulation time for blood clotting
♦ Increases urea and fluid secretion
♦ Stimulates and brightens the mind
♦ Controls and regulates body fat
♦ Controls intestinal activity
♦ Aids the function of the pancreas
♦ Helps to harmonize the activity of the adrenal glands
♦ Has a regulating influence on the ovaries and testicles
♦ Works in cooperation with the parathyroid, thereby regulating the action of mineral salts in the system, especially of calcium
♦ Acts in conjunction with the pituitary gland

Lecithin

Lecithin is found in every cell or organ in the body. It is also necessary to every cell and organ. Theoretically, by eating it in sufficient amounts, you can help rebuild those cells or organs which need it. Once they are repaired, the lecithin helps to maintain their health. To date, there is a mounting accumulation of scientific studies which suggest some of the diverse benefits of lecithin.

♦ Lecithin has been found to reduce blood cholesterol levels in some individuals
♦ It helps dissolve the plaques in the arteries, in some cases
♦ It also has been noted as valuable in eliminating the yellow or yellow-brown plaque on the skin or around the eyes caused by fatty deposits
♦ Lecithin helps lower the blood pressure in some people
♦ It produces greater alertness in elderly people
♦ It increases the gamma globulin in the blood which helps fight infection
♦ Lecithin benefits certain skin disturbances, including eczema, acne, and psoriasis
♦ It fills out and softens aging skin where dryness, paper-thinness and shriveling occur
♦ Lecithin has been used to restore sexual powers and glandular exhaustion; seminal fluid is rich in lecithin, and because of its loss from the body, men's need for it may be especially great
♦ Lecithin helps in the assimilation of vitamins A and E
♦ It lengthens the lives of animals, producing glossier coats and greater alertness
♦ Lecithin, with the additional help of vitamin E, has been found to lower the requirements of insulin in some cases of diabetes

Liver

Liver, usually calf liver or beef liver:

♦ Has an anti-anemia factor
♦ Has a growth factor

- ◆ Has an energy metabolism factor which resists muscular fatigue
- ◆ Has an anti-estrogen factor
- ◆ Contains a high percentage of protein
- ◆ Is packed with many valuable vitamins, minerals and amino acids

Liver is in some ways a near-perfect food, but if you do not like liver, or don't eat it frequently, don't worry. A perfect substitute is desiccated liver, which is available in tablet or powder form.

The down side of liver is that, since it is the organ that detoxifies and eliminates poisons, animals which are given drugs, hormones and pesticide-laced feed (this includes most chickens and beef), may have a higher concentration of these pollutants in their livers than anywhere else in the body except the fatty tissues. If you do eat liver or take the tablets, be sure it comes from a pure source. Look for "range-fed" chickens and hormone-free beef.

Papaya, the "Magic Melon"

The tropical fruit papaya:

- ◆ Can prevent your stomach from being queasy
- ◆ Helps digestion
- ◆ Digests 2,230 times its own weight in starch
- ◆ Tenderizes meat

In today's hurried world, we grab, gorge and overindulge. Unfortunately, our stomachs were not made to take that kind of abuse. What is the usual remedy we run for? You guessed it: antacids that fizzle and sizzle like seltzer and taste like chalk. We down chemicals disguised as candy or mints, or we swallow chalky liquids. There is a natural way to counteract overindulgence. That remedy is Nature's own papaya. You can eat this delicious fruit fresh, or take papaya enzyme

71

tablets, which can actually digest 2,230 times their weight of starch.

How can papaya do this? Simple. It contains the natural enzymes papain and prolase. These two enzymes assist in protein digestion and combine with mylase, a potent starch-digestive enzyme. The best way to take your papaya is after each meal. Papain is the chief ingredient in meat tenderizers that work on fowl, fish and beef before reaching your stomach.

Pectin

Does pectin lower cholesterol?

Research conducted by Dr. Hans Fisher, Chairman of the Department of Nutrition at Rutgers University, clearly shows that pectin "limits the amount of cholesterol the body can absorb." Dr. Fisher and his associates were quoted as saying that pectin, which is a natural carbohydrate found in fruits and vegetables, "offers partial protection" against the dangerous health problems associated with elevated cholesterol. Pectin showed its ability to lower serum cholesterol levels in various animals and humans. Dr. Fisher reported that college students taking 10 grams of pectin per day for three weeks experienced roughly a 20 percent reduction in average cholesterol levels.

According to the British medical journal Lancet, A. S. Turswell and Ruth M. Kay of Queen Elizabeth College's Nutrition Department in London, gave 15 grams of citrus pectin daily in divided doses to three subjects. All showed reduction in cholesterol levels averaging 15 percent.

Ten to 15 grams of pectin a day represents about three to six whole apples. Fortunately, pectin is available in concentrated form in tablets. The old adage of "an apple a day" seems more true today than ever before.

♦ Helps prevent heart trouble (with wheat germ)
♦ Helps dissolve gallstones
♦ Helps reverse gout
♦ Helps the aches and stabbing pains of neuritis
♦ Helps cancer patients subjected to heavy radiation (given yeast daily, some patients did not suffer from the anemia and vomiting which occurred in patients not protected by yeast)

Yeast is an excellent source of protein and a superior source of the B-complex vitamins. It is one of the richest providers of organic iron as well as most other minerals and trace minerals and amino acids. It stimulates energy and relieves fatigue, constipation, nervousness and indigestion. It is also a perfect reducing food. Yeast helps lower cholesterol (when combined with lecithin), corrects cirrhosis of the liver by rejuvenating the liver, and clears eczema (also acne).

There are various sources of yeast:

brewer's yeast (from hops, a byproduct of beer), sometimes called nutritional yeast,

torula yeast, grown on wood pulp used in the manufacture of paper, or from blackstrap molasses;

whey, byproduct of milk and cheese (best tasting and most potent);

liquid yeast from Switzerland and Germany, fed on herbs, honey, malt and oranges or grapefruit.

Avoid live baker's yeast. Live yeast cells are vitamin robbers, especially of B vitamins in the intestines. In nutritional yeast, these live cells are heat killed, and thus are prevented from stealing B vitamins from your body. Yeast has all the major B vitamins except B12, which can be especially bred into it; it contains 16 amino acids, 14 or more minerals and 17 vitamins (though not A, E or C). Yeast can be considered a whole food. Because yeast, like other protein food, is high in phosphorus, it is advisable when taking it to add extra calcium to the diet. Phosphorus, a coworker of calcium, can take calcium out of the body with it, leaving a calcium deficiency. The remedy is simple: Take extra calcium (calcium lactate assimilates well in the body). The B complex should be taken with yeast to be more effective. Together they work like a powerhouse.

Yeast can be stirred into liquid, juice or water and taken between meals. Many people who feel fatigued take a tablespoon or more in liquid and feel a return of energy within minutes, and the good effects last for several hours.

The Roles of Protein, Amino Acids, Lipotropics and Enzymes in Nutrition

Protein

- ♦ Supplies the body with energy
- ♦ Is necessary for growth in children
- ♦ Is necessary for adults to maintain their body structure
- ♦ Every cell in your body contains protein

Protein is the basic nutrient capable of building, repairing and maintaining all the body tissues. Protein is the master builder of the human body. It is the most complex substance known to man. Protein contains nitrogen and sulfur which break up or oxidize to obtain energy.

Foods highest in protein are:
1. meat, fish
2. eggs
3. cheese made from milk
4. lentils, soybeans
5. nuts
6. oats, sweet potatoes (high-quality protein)

Amino Acids

There are many components of protein, called amino acids. Only some amino acids are produced in the body. The others must be supplied from food intake; these are called the "essential" amino acids. An * indicates that this is an essential amino acid.

The branched-chain amino acids (leucine, isoleucine and valine), also called BCAAs, can reduce the appetite while preserving basic protein storage in the body. Some 15 to 20 percent of muscle is composed of BCAAs. In one hour, 50 percent of ingested BCAAs goes to your muscles; 100 percent in two hours. BCAAs promote lean muscle distribution and are anabolic, meaning they build up muscle tissue. BCAAs produce glycogen, which helps balance insulin secretion.

All amino acids should be taken in between meals with juice or water—not with protein.

ALANINE
Enhances the immune system, lowers the risk of kidney stones, and aids in alleviating hypoglycemia by regulating sugar metabolism.

ARGININE
Increases the sperm content in the male, accelerates wound healing, tones muscle tissue, helps metabolize stored body fat, and promotes physical and mental alertness.

ASPARTIC ACID (NOT AVAILABLE IN THE USA)
Enhances the immune system, increases stamina and endurance, expels harmful ammonia from the body.

CARNITINE
Used by athletes, permitting longer periods of intense workouts, converts stored body fat into energy, can control hypoglycemia, reduce angina attacks and

benefit diabetics, and liver and kidney disease; deficiency can cause impairment of heart tissue.

CITRULLINE

Helps recovery from fatigue, stimulates the immune system, metabolizes to arginine, and detoxifies ammonia, which is poisonous to cells.

CYSTINE, CYSTEINE*

- ♦ Cysteine is an important antiaging nutrient
- ♦ Cystine and cysteine can be readily converted by the body into one another
- ♦ Help to detoxify the system
- ♦ Protect against copper toxicity
- ♦ Are antioxidants (free-radical fighters)
- ♦ Can protect against X-ray and nuclear radiation

D, L PHENYLALANINE

Acts as a natural painkiller, selectively blocks pain, and is nonaddictive. It is an effective pain reliever for whiplash, osteoarthritis, rheumatoid arthritis, lower back pain, nighttime muscle and leg cramps, and postoperative pain. It is also an antidepressant.

GAMMA-BUTYRIC ACID (GABA)

One of the best-known substances that transmit nerve impulses to the brain (a neurotransmitter). It may be involved with the release of growth hormone.

GLUTAMIC ACID AND GLUTAMINE

Helps improve brain function, alleviates fatigue, aids in ulcer healing time, acts as a mood elevator, may serve as a brain stimulant. It provides Y-butyric amino acid.

GLUTATHIONE

An antiaging agent, synthesized from three amino acids—cysteine, glutamic acid and clycine—antitumor agent, respiratory accelerator in the brain, helps prevent harmful side effects of high-dose radiation, chemotherapy and X-rays.

GLYCINE
Produces glycogen, which mobilizes glucose (blood sugar) from the liver, bolsters the immune system, effective against hyperacidity. Serves as a stimulant to the brain. It also aids in healing of swollen and infected prostate.

HISTIDINE
Precursor of histamine. Helps keep people from biting their nails, dilates blood vessels, helps alleviate symptoms of rheumatoid arthritis, alleviates stress, aids in improving libido.

ISOLEUCINE*
Needed in hemoglobin formation.

L-PHENYLALANINE
Improves memory and mental alertness, acts as an antidepressant, helps suppress appetite, increases sexual interest.

LEUCINE*
It is found to be lacking in alcoholics and drug addicts, as are three other amino acids, L-glutamine, A-amino-n-butyric acid and citrulline.

LYSINE*
Deficiency may cause nausea, dizziness and anemia. Helps improve concentration, enhances fertility, aids in preventing fever blisters or cold sores (herpes simplex) and shortening the healing period for herpes. L-lysine monohydrochloride builds new body tissue and also such vital substances as antibodies, hormones, enzymes and body cells. Lysine is found in meat, eggs, fish, milk and cheese.

METHIONINE
Lipotropic agent, reduces fat and protects the kidney, aids in lowering cholesterol, natural chelating

agent for heavy metals. Aids in producing beautiful skin. Methionine can be substituted for choline, which aids in reducing liver fat (lipotropic agent) and protects the kidneys. It also builds new bony tissue. A deficiency of methionine may lead to fatty degeneration and cirrhosis of the liver. Methionine can be found in meat, eggs, fish, milk and cheese.

ORNITHINE
Works as a muscle-building substance, increases potency of arginine.

PHENYLALANINE*
Cannot be metabolized if a person is deficient in vitamin C. It is a stimulant which sends impulses to the brain, acts as an antidepressant and can raise blood pressure.

PROLINE
Aids in wound healing, helps increase learning ability.

SERINE
Helps alleviate pain, produces cellular energy, is a natural antipsychotic, converts to cystine in the body.

TAURINE
Used to treat some forms of epilepsy by controlling seizures; found in high concentration in the tissues of the heart, skeletal muscle and central nervous system.

THREONINE*
Low in vegetarian diets, essential to normal growth, helps prevent fatty buildup in liver, necessary for utilization of protein in the diet. Deficiency results in negative hydrogen balance in the body.

TRYPTOPHAN (NOT AVAILABLE IN THE USA AT THIS TIME)
Provides niacin, which prevents pellagra and mental

deficiency. It regulate sleep. A deficiency causes insomnia. It is useful as a relaxant as well.

Tryptophan was widely used as a sleep aid until a contaminated batch out of Japan killed eleven people. Unfortunately, in spite of the fact that tryptophan is safe and is used in baby foods and nutritional powders for senior citizens, the FDA has pulled it off the market as a nutritional supplement as of this writing. Tryptophan is a wonderful amino acid that aids in reducing anxiety, helps induce sleep and may help in alcoholism.

TYROSINE

Acts in regulation of emotional behavior. Important in eventual synthesis of thyroxine, thus aiding in prevention of hypothyroidism. It also yields L-dopa, which has a side effect of increasing sexuality. Phenylalanine converts to tyrosine. It has an important role in stimulating and modifying brain activity, helps control drug-resistant depression and anxiety, as well as helping amphetamine takers to reduce their dosage to minimal levels in a few weeks. It can also help cocaine addicts kick their habit, by helping to avert the depression, fatigue and extreme irritability which accompany withdrawal.

VALINE

A deficiency results in negative hydrogen balance in the body.

The Lipotropics

Lipotropics are substances that prevent an abnormal accumulation of fat in the liver. The four lipotropics are methionine, choline, inositol and betaine. What do the lipotropics do exactly?

1. They increase production of lecithin by the liver. This helps to keep cholesterol more soluble, thereby lessening cholesterol deposits in blood vessels and also lessening the chances of gallstone formation. (Gall-stones usually have a large component of cholesterol.)

2. They prevent accumulation of fats in the liver.

Fatty liver is probably the main reason for sluggish liver function. Methionine seems to act as a catalyst for choline and inositol, speeding up their function.

3. They detoxify the liver.

Methionine and choline detoxify amines, which are byproducts of protein metabolism. This is especially important for persons on a high-protein diet.

4. They increase resistance to disease.

Lipotropics help to increase resistance to disease by bolstering the thymus gland in carrying out its antidisease function in three ways:

♦ By stimulating the production of antibodies
♦ By stimulating the growth and action of phago-cytes, which surround and gobble up invading viruses and microbes
♦ By recognizing and destroying foreign and abnormal tissue

Enzymes

Enzymes are complex proteins necessary for the digestion of food. They release valuable vitamins, minerals and amino acids which keep us alive and healthy. Enzymes are catalysts, i.e., they have the power to cause an internal action without changing or destroying themselves in the process. Each enzyme acts upon a specific food; one cannot substitute for another. A shortage or deficiency, or even the absence of one single enzyme, can make all the difference between health and sickness.

Because enzymes are destroyed when they are heated, uncooked or unprocessed fruits and vegetables are excellent sources. Raw meat, fish and eggs are also good sources of enzymes, but can't be recommended because of contamination by parasites and bacteria, which heating kills.

Pepsin is a vital digestive enzyme which breaks up the proteins of ingested food, splitting them into usable amino acids. Without pepsin, protein could not be used to build healthy skin, strong skeletal structure, rich blood supply and strong muscles.

Renin is a digestive enzyme which causes coagulation of milk, changing its protein, casein, into a usable form in the body. Renin releases the valuable minerals in milk—calcium, phosphorus, potassium and iron—which are used by the body to stabilize the water balance, strengthen the nervous system and produce strong teeth and bones.

Lipase splits fat, which is then utilized to nourish the skin cells, protect the body against bruises and blows, and ward off the entrance of infectious virus cells and allergic conditions.

Hydrochloric acid (HCl) is a digestive acid secreted in normal stomachs. It digests protein, calcium, and iron. Hydrochloric acid in the stomach works on tough foods such as fibrous meats, vegetables, and poultry. A deficiency of HCl in the stomach can cause improper digestion as well as loss of valuable vitamins and minerals. After watching all those television commercials, you are probably saying to yourself that you don't need any more acid since you have heartburn and are taking an antacid. In fact, you may have exactly the opposite problem. Since the symptoms of too little acid are just the same as too much acid, the taking of antacids could be the worst possible thing to do.

The best way to discover whether you need HCl supplementation or not is to take an HCl tablet with betaine plus pepsin after a protein meal. If that "lump feeling" or gas remains, you may have too much acid, which is rare indeed. To overcome this burning sensation, drink a glass of water, which flushes away the excess HCl.

"The rat race," stress, tension, anger and worry before eating can all cause a lack of HCl. Deficiencies of some vitamins (B complex primarily) and minerals can also cause a lack of HCl. Most of us eat too quickly and do not allow our systems to digest food correctly. People with flatulence (gas) can cause the condition themselves by gulping down food and inhaling air too quickly. To sum up, if I may borrow an old television commercial slogan: "Try HCl; you'll like it."

Modern Maladies

PROSTATE TROUBLES

Over 20 percent of all American men over the age of 50 will develop prostate problems of some kind, and one in eleven will develop prostate cancer. By the time we are 70, over 50 percent of us will have an enlarged prostate gland, and by the time we are 80, the number goes up to 85 percent. A high-fat diet, low zinc levels and an imbalance of male hormones in the gland appear to be the major causes of prostate troubles. What "modern" medicine has to offer you if you have prostate troubles are drugs and surgery that are only sometimes effective and often have side effects such as impotence and urinary dysfunction. (For surgery these side effects are permanent.)

The prostate is a gland in men located at the neck of the bladder and urethra (the tube through which urine and semen pass on the way out of the body). It's about the size and shape of a chestnut in an adult male.

The prostate stays about the same size until we reach the age when some male hormones begin to decline (in most men, their fifties), and the prostate begins to grow again. If the gland grows too much, it begins to pinch the urethra, interfering with urination. Symptoms of an enlarged prostate—benign prostatic hypertrophy (BPH)—can include dribbling, a decrease in the size of the stream during urination, frequent or difficult urination, and chronic discomfort in the abdominal area.

Some scientists believe that when testosterone production declines, other male hormones synthesized from testosterone not only decline but are thrown out of balance, causing prostate enlargement. Unfortunately the answer is not as simple as giving men testosterone supplementation—we learned the hard way that this not only causes the prostate to enlarge even more but can also cause the growth of prostate tumors.

Testosterone also regulates the production of prostaglandins, which seem to keep prostate growth under control. Foods that support the production of prostaglandins contain essential fatty acids (EFAs) such as the omega-3 oils found mainly in fish.

Many studies suggest that a high-fat diet is a major culprit in prostate troubles in men. Among Japanese men, who traditionally eat a diet low in fat and high in soy products, prostate problems are rare, as they are in other cultures that favor low-fat diets. However, a study of Japanese men who moved to Hawaii and presumably began eating a typically high-fat American diet, showed that they had prostate problems at the same rate as Americans. A study of 51,000 American men, ages 40–75, who were followed for two to four years, showed that prostate cancer was directly related to total fat consumption, with red meat showing the strongest association with advanced cancer. Another study in Italy comparing 271 men with prostate cancer to 685 men who did not have the disease concluded that a high dietary consumption of milk was a significant indicator of prostate cancer risk, even in men who also ate a lot of whole grains and fresh vegetables.

Other studies have linked prostate cancer to exposure to herbicides used in agriculture, forestry and in cities and suburbs to control weeds.

Vitamins that Are Good for the Prostate

Zinc is necessary for the proper function of the prostate gland. In men, higher concentrations of this mineral are found in the prostate than anywhere else in the body. A recent study looked at zinc supplementation in young men and found that when plasma zinc levels were low, there was a corresponding drop in testosterone. There have been many clinical studies showing that zinc supplementation can reduce the size of the prostate gland, along with troublesome symptoms.

I recommend that all men take up to 30 to 50 mg (not more than 50, please) of zinc daily, and include zinc-rich foods in the diet such as oysters (well-cooked, please!), lamb chops and wheat germ. Pumpkin seeds are a good source of zinc, and are also rich in the amino acids alanine, glycine and glutamic acid, which seem to have a positive effect in reducing the size of the prostate. A handful of dried pumpkin seeds a day is plenty.

Selenium is another important mineral in male hormone regulation that is found in large amounts in the prostate. Blood levels of both zinc and selenium are low in men who have prostate cancer. Men who live in areas where the soil is rich in selenium tend to have lower rates of prostate cancer. Rich sources of selenium are garlic, shellfish, grains and chicken. If you're over the age of 50, I suggest you supplement your diet with up to 200 mcg of selenium daily. Please do not exceed this amount, as it can be toxic in high doses.

Soy products such as miso, tofu and tempeh may help reduce the risk of prostate enlargement and cancer. The Japanese diet, which is heavy in soy products, may be protective against prostate enlargement and tumors.

Saw Palmetto

As I mention in my book *Earl Mindell's Herb Bible*, an extract made from the berry of saw palmetto *(Serenoa repens)* also called sabal, a palm tree native to Florida, Texas and Georgia, has been shown in numerous studies to reduce the urinary symptoms caused by prostate enlargement. Although the exact action of saw palmetto hasn't been pinpointed, it is theorized that it inhibits the production of a hormone that affects the prostate. You can find saw palmetto in your health food store in capsules or tincture form.

A Healthy Prostate Diet

Eat More

Fish oils or other sources of omega-3 fatty acids

Soy products such as soybeans, miso, tofu and tempeh

Fiber

Drink More

Clean water (at least 6–8 glasses daily)

Avoid

Red meat

Whole milk (yogurt is OK)

Processed vegetable oils

Other foods sources that can support your prostate:

Daily

Wheat germ

A handful of pumpkin seeds

Garlic daily as a supplement or food

Weekly

Hormone-free chicken (a good source of selenium)

Oysters or lamb chops every other week (a good source of zinc)

Supplements

Zinc: 20–50 mg daily

Selenium: 100–200 mcg daily

Herbs

Saw palmetto: 2 capsules 3 times daily, or 20–40 drops daily, or follow directions on the bottle, or ask your alternative health care professional.

BREAST CANCER

Breast cancer is the most common form of cancer in American women, with about 150,000 new cases diagnosed each year. It is the second most common cause of death from cancer after lung cancer, claiming approximately 50,000 lives each year. The average American woman has a one-in-nine chance of developing breast cancer in her lifetime. (Since the chance of getting breast cancer goes way up as women age, the one-in-nine figure represents an average. In other words, the chance of a 30-year-old woman getting breast cancer is *much* lower than that of a 70-year-old woman. This is still a very sobering statistic.)

There *are* simple steps you can take to reduce your risk of getting breast cancer.

Cut the Fat

Cutting down on the fat in your diet, particularly animal fat, is the single most important step that you can take, not only in preventing breast cancer, but in improving your overall health. You will also be protecting yourself from heart disease, the number-one killer of women in the United States.

There is evidence linking breast cancer with high

levels of animal fat in the diet. Please cut down on it. Another issue in breast cancer is estrogen. Breast tissue in premenopausal women gets a monthly influx of reproductive hormones, estrogen among them, making it a more inviting environment for cancer cells than most other fatty tissue—estrogen encourages cell reproduction, and that includes cancer cells. Fat is intimately linked to the amount of the reproductive hormone estrogen circulating in the body: The more fat in the diet, the more estrogen in the blood. The more estrogen in the blood through a woman's lifetime, the higher the rate of breast cancer. Even body fat produces estrogens, so the more fat on your body, the higher the level of circulating estrogens.

Once a woman goes through menopause, her risk of breast cancer increases, so please don't add ERT (estrogen replacement therapy) on top of this unless you are among the very small percentage of women who are actually low in estrogen.

In a study done of 14,290 women between 1985 and 1991 by New York University, it was found that concentrations of DDT were 35 percent higher in women with cancer. Cancer patients also have higher levels of PCBs and dioxins, byproducts of manufacturing that contaminate our water supply and fish, and our food supply. Avoid any unnecessary exposure to chemicals, drugs and other potential environmental carcinogens.

Here are a few more tips for preventing breast cancer:

♦ Take vitamin C daily. It's a powerful antioxidant, a substance which cleans harmful substances out of cells.
♦ Take vitamin E daily. It's another powerful antioxidant.
♦ Take beta carotene, a form of vitamin A, daily. Beta carotene is another powerful antioxidant

which has shown up again and again in studies as a cancer preventive. In the most recent study, the *New England Journal of Medicine* reported that women whose diets were low in vitamin A were at a 20 percent higher risk of breast cancer. Good food sources of beta carotene include carrots, spinach, sweet potatoes, cantaloupes and yellow squash.

♦ Take a vitamin B complex. The B vitamins will help your liver get rid of excess estrogen.

♦ Drink lots of clean water and eat plenty of fiber—water is Nature's best body cleanser, inside and out. By drinking plenty of clean water every day you are assisting your body in ridding itself of toxins. Fiber is Nature's second-best inner cleanser, pushing food speedily through the digestive system, taking with it toxins and impurities.

COLON CANCER

Colon cancer is a topic most people prefer to avoid, but 57,000 people will die of it this year. This is tragic, because so many colon cancers can be prevented so easily. The accuracy levels for detecting early colon cancer are not very high, and if you don't detect it early you have a good chance of dying from it. So let's talk about preventing colon cancer in the first place!

We know you can have a genetic predisposition to get colon cancer, and we also know two major factors that can cause colon cancer:

♦ There are a lot of toxic substances passing through your system that will harm your bowel, and possibly create cancerous cells, if they sit there for very long.

♦ Many studies have linked a high-fat diet to colon cancer. Fat stimulates your gall bladder to produce bile, which is one of those toxic substances that shouldn't sit there. Also, the high temperatures needed to cook fat can produce potentially cancer-causing substances in your food.

♦ It is also significant that low levels of the mineral selenium have been repeatedly linked to colon cancer.

Five Tips for Preventing Colon Cancer

1) **Keep things moving through your bowels.** Chow down on vegetables such as broccoli, kale, carrots, onions, cabbage, collards, peas, potatoes and all dark green, yellow and orange vegetables. They're high in fiber so they keep your bowels moving, but that's not all. They contain substances that take toxins through your intestines quickly and harmlessly. And don't forget the wheat bran for more fiber. There is some evidence that fiber may even reverse the growth of precancerous polyps (bumps or growths in the lining of your intestines). The seeds of psyllium, a kind of plantain, are the best source of fiber, before fruits and vegetables and beans. Just a tablespoon a day with two glasses of water will be effective.

2) **Cut down on the saturated fat** you're eating. Saturated fat is usually solid at room temperature. Examples are butter, the marbled fat in meat, the fat from fried foods, and hydrogenated oils. Cut your fat consumption to 20 percent or less of your caloric intake. Of that 20 percent, be sure that only 10 percent or less comes from saturated fat.

3) **Get your calcium**—it is paramount in the prevention of colon cancer. The French eat five to six servings of yogurt daily, and even though they consume

as much fat as most North Americans, their rate of colon cancer is much lower.

4) **Take your selenium!** Over the past few years a number of studies have linked low selenium levels with colon cancer, but researchers didn't know whether that was a cause or an effect of the disease. In a more recent study at the University of Arizona, it was found that people with high levels of selenium in their blood had fewer colon polyps, which are often precancerous.

Onion and garlic are rich sources of selenium, which is an important part of an antioxidant enzyme called glutathione peroxidase. This enzyme may prevent damage to cells. Some studies show that it plays a role in the repair of DNA and helps activate the immune system. If you take selenium supplements, do not take more than 100 to 200 mcg daily. Other great sources of selenium are seafood, kidney, liver, wheat germ, bran, tuna fish, tomatoes and broccoli.

5) **Exercise! Exercise! Exercise!** The more you exercise, the faster your food moves through your digestive system.

CONSTIPATION

If you aren't constipated yourself, you probably know someone who is. About 30 million Americans are afflicted with this uncomfortable and unhealthy problem. So why aren't America's bowels moving? We need to eat more fiber, drink more water and get more exercise. Whatever you do, avoid those habit-forming over-the-counter laxatives.

Whole-grain breads and cereals contain fiber, which helps food move easily through our digestive tract. Fiber also has the added benefit of lowering cholesterol. Fresh fruits, vegetables and legumes (beans) also contain fiber.

The best all-around fiber laxative is bran. You'll get

bran naturally if you eat whole grains. There are many cereals in the supermarket with bran in them. You can buy bran in a jar and sprinkle it on your cereal or in your yogurt—try starting with a heaping tablespoon. Wheat bran is the most common bran in America, but rice and corn bran also work well to relieve constipation. Prunes work wonders for many people with constipation. Have three or four for breakfast and see what happens. Popcorn is a good laxative for some people.

It's important not to introduce too much fiber or "roughage" into your diet too quickly. If you do, you may suffer from bloating, gas and abdominal cramps. Gradually introduce more whole grains, more fresh fruits and vegetables, and more water to your diet. If you're not getting some exercise every day, add that too. Give it three weeks. If that doesn't work, try bran or prunes. Start with a heaping tablespoon of bran and then gradually add more if you need to.

Water naturally softens stools. If you are taking a diuretic medicine, it will tend to pull water out of your bowels, and can cause constipation. Please drink 7–10 glasses of clean water every day. Coffee can help move your bowels unless you overdo it. Drink too much coffee and you may end up constipated.

Some pharmaceutical drugs cause constipation, including pain killers, decongestants, narcotics, antihistamines, antidepressants and tranquilizers. Iron tablets can cause constipation.

If you try the above remedies and you're still constipated, try psyllium powder. It's made from a fibrous plant that can help give your stools more bulk. It's the main ingredient in products such as Metamucil, but you can get it in a much purer and cheaper form at your local health food store. Mix about a teaspoon with apple juice and drink right away. It's very important to drink plenty of fluids when you're using a bulk-forming laxative such as psyllium.

Herbs such as cascara sagrada and senna can relieve constipation by stimulating the bowels. In general I don't recommend them because they can become habit-forming, but once in a while they are fine. Cascara sagrada is made from the bark of a tree, and is fairly gentle. It is found in some over-the-counter laxatives, but I suggest you get it in capsule form at your local health food store.

Senna is another plant laxative. It is a more powerfully bowel-stimulating laxative that has been commonly used for centuries. Stimulating laxatives become habit-forming if your bowels lose their natural ability to be stimulated. Try to use them only when absolutely necessary.

STRESS

Stress is one of the worst modern maladies. In today's tense world, stress can cause diseases such as ulcers, colitis and high blood pressure. In fact, it has been stated that 75 percent of the patients of a general-practice physician have some symptoms caused by emotionally induced illness. It is interesting to note that the weakest part of the human anatomy is the gastrointestinal tract (the gut).

It has been proven that during times of stress, the body's need for certain nutrients is greatly increased. Increased tension and stress are usually accompanied by inability to sleep, loss or gain of weight, exhaustion, irritability, depression and loss of emotional control, as well as numerous aches and pains, either slight or severe.

Pituitary and adrenal hormones are the body's way of counteracting prolonged stress. This is where nutrition begins to play a very significant role. Vitamin E, pantothenic acid and the remainder of the B-complex vitamins are necessary for the proper functioning of the pituitary and adrenal glands. Vitamin C need during stress is increased greatly because it accelerates the rate of cortisone production. Also, vitamin C may be the detoxifying agent the body needs during stress conditions.

Here are some tips for beating stress:

Avoid

Junk food. During a stressful period, throw away your candy bars, potato chips and coffee, and reach for protein.

Too much coffee. More than 2 or 3 cups will make you jittery, deplete your adrenal glands and rob you of needed vitamins and minerals.

Sugar. It can pick up your energy for a short time, but you're likely to feel even lower as little as a half hour later. If you're craving something sweet, try fruit, which contains a lot of sugar, but in a form better tolerated by the body.

Excess alcohol. Alcohol may be a relaxant for some, but it also pulls vitamins and minerals out of the body and can leave the mind and body feeling dull the next morning.

Too much animal fat. Animal fat can provide an energy boost, but too much will tax your liver, which is already stressed out when you're stressed out. A small serving of meat with lunch or dinner can give your body a nutritional boost, but too much will bring it down.

Fried food. By all means avoid French fries and other fried foods, which are generally made with rancid vegetable oils! Rancid oil is full of free radicals which cause cell damage, and it's very hard on your liver, which is already working hard enough to keep your body free of toxins.

HIGH CHOLESTEROL

Cholesterol is a fatlike substance used in many of the body's chemical processes. To maintain good health, our bodies require a certain amount of cholesterol.

What we don't need is an elevated serum cholesterol level, which too many of us have. Excess cholesterol that cannot be utilized by the body enters your bloodstream. Cholesterol deposits can build up on the coronary arteries. Slowly but steadily, year after year, this buildup continues. The outcome is artery walls thickened by plaquelike deposits. Less blood and oxygen can be delivered to the heart muscle. Thus the heart has to work harder. A heart attack may occur if the blockage in the artery becomes severe enough.

As much as possible, try to reduce your intake of foods high in cholesterol or containing saturated fats—these fats seem to contribute most to high cholesterol levels.

Many physicians recommend the following steps to reduce your risk of a heart attack:

♦ Replace saturated fats with polyunsaturated fats whenever possible
♦ Keep your weight at normal levels
♦ Stop smoking
♦ Avoid stress
♦ Exercise regularly
♦ Have regular checkups

INSOMNIA

VALERIAN
Sometimes at the end of a long day I'm "wired but tired." My body is telling me it's time to sleep, but my mind is keeping me awake. When that happens I take a dropperful of valerian tincture in water, and within 30 minutes I'm fast asleep. Valerian (*Valeriana officinalis L.*) is a plant that has been used for thousands of years as a folk remedy for "nervous stomach" and as a sedative. Valerian has few if any side effects and is not habit-forming. Although valerian is available

in capsule form, it's best taken as a tincture (a fluid extract of the herb, suspended in alcohol or glycerine).

CALCIUM AND MAGNESIUM
When your grandmother gave you a glass of milk before bedtime, she was wisely giving you a dose of calcium to relax your muscles and ease you into sleep. Magnesium regulates calcium uptake by cells, so take a magnesium/calcium combination for the greatest effect. Two tablets of 600 mg calcium/300 mg magnesium will give you sweet dreams.

EXERCISE
Exercise is one of the best sleep aids around. Am I suggesting you get up in the middle of the night and run around the block? No way! I am suggesting that if you've taken a brisk walk or gotten some other kind of exercise during the day, you'll sleep better and wake up more refreshed.

WHAT TO AVOID
Caffeine and alcohol are two of sleep's biggest enemies. We all know that coffee can keep you awake, but alcohol? Yes, it's a muscle relaxant, but too much alcohol can actually keep you awake. It also causes sleep pattern disturbances, depletes your body of vitamins and minerals, and acts as a diuretic, so you wake up feeling groggy and thirsty.

I hope I don't need to tell you to avoid sleeping pills like the plague! Most of them have unpleasant side effects, are habit-forming, and leave you groggy in the morning. Some even suppress REM or dream sleep, which can leave you feeling mentally out of it the next day.

Should you eat right before you go to sleep? Some people say it gives them nightmares, and others say it helps sleep better. This is very individual, and depends on your blood sugar, your digestion and your metabolism. However, if you do eat before bed, stick to simple foods like a piece of toast, a bowl of cereal (no sugar, whole grains please), fruit (bananas work well) or crackers (low-salt, whole-grain). Avoid white sugar, spicy foods and fat—they can keep you awake and be hard to digest.

Nutrition for Special Needs

NUTRITION FOR TRAVELERS

The average American family saves for 50 weeks a year to go on a two-week vacation. A great deal of planning and expense goes into that two or three-week or even month-long trip. If you are planning a trip to Europe, Mexico, or the Orient, a few words about nutrition can help you to have a healthier experience.

In Europe, a continental breakfast supplies you with rolls, coffee and marmalade. This meal was not designed to promote energy production, nor are late European dinners conducive to early-morning appetites. Try to add more protein and less fat and white flour to your European breakfasts!

A good multivitamin-mineral supplement with a complete B complex is essential. B vitamins are available in brewer's yeast and liver tablets. Vitamin C is also very important. Five hundred-milligram tablets are the most convenient. For travelers on a hectic schedule (if it's Tuesday, this must be Belgium) antistress B complex with at least 200 mg of pantothenic acid might come in handy.

In Asian countries, where protein is not prominent in the diet, a pep-up protein powder added to your juice in the morning will give you extra energy. If possible, eat yogurt on your vacation. The friendly bacteria can help to prevent dysentery. Yogurt is also available in concentrated tablet form. The yogurt bacteria break milk sugar into lactic acid and discourage the growth of pathogenic organisms. Two or three yogurt tablets a day, seven days before your vacation and during it, give the best results.

Remember, you are paying a lot for your vacation; you might as well enjoy it in the best of health. Have a great time!

NUTRITION FOR HEALTHY SKIN AND HAIR

Shiny, lustrous hair is a sign of good health. If your hair isn't as healthy as you'd like it to be, a few supplements can help a lot. When we aren't getting the nutrients we need, our hair will show it by being dull and brittle.

Healthy Hair Vitamins, Minerals and Supplements

Be sure these nutrients are a daily part of your diet:

Protein. Meat, fish, poultry, legumes combined with grains, soy products.

Vitamin A. Liver, egg yolks, nonfat milk, yellow and orange vegetables and fruits, dark green leafy vegetables.

Vitamin E (tocopherol). Olive oil, whole grains, avocado, nuts

Iodine. Seafood, iodized salt, kelp.

Iron. Meat is the best source of iron.

Cysteine. An amino acid found in large amounts in the hair. Eggs, meat and dairy products are good sources of cysteine. You can also take cysteine capsules. If you are diabetic or allergic to monosodium glutamate, do not take cysteine.

Biotin. Although a biotin deficiency is rare, it can cause hair loss and dry skin. Biotin can be depleted by low-calorie weight-loss diets, oral antibiotics and a steady diet of raw egg whites. Eating foods high in biotin—nuts, whole grains, organ meats such as liver, and vegetables—can reverse hair loss caused by a biotin deficiency. Although there is no scientific evidence that they work, some people swear by shampoo and conditioning products with biotin in them.

Thyroid. Dull, lifeless hair can be caused by a thyroid deficiency. Iodine is important for proper thyroid metabolism. It's found naturally in fish, and is added to most table salt. Check with your physician if you have reason to believe you are hypothyroid.

Other Healthy Hair Tips:

♦ Wash your hair in lukewarm water, and rinse it in cool water.
♦ Use shampoos with natural ingredients—check your health food store.
♦ Protect your hair from the sun and wind, which will dry it.
♦ Wear a bathing cap when swimming in chlorinated pools.
♦ Rinse your hair right away after swimming in the ocean.
♦ If possible, avoid or go easy on hair dyes (most of them contain coal tar, which is carcinogenic), bleaches and perms. They will all eventually make your hair dull.
♦ The constant use of hot combs, heated rollers and blow dryers can also make your hair dull.
♦ Dry your hair by wrapping it in a towel rather than rubbing it.

My Basic Vitamin-Mineral Program
for Beginners

Not everyone requires the same vitamins and minerals. Here's a basic program. Ideally you'll take a high-potency multiple vitamin supplement at least twice a day that gives you:

- Beta carotene, 10-25,000 IU
- B complex, 50-75 mg each of B1, B2, B6, PABA, pantothenic acid, folic acid, biotin, B12, choline, inositol, niacinamide
- Vitamin D, 400 IU
- Vitamin C complex 500–1,000 mg (with bioflavonoids)
- Vitamin E, 400 IU
- High-potency multiple mineral mix of:
  calcium 600 mg
  magnesium 300 mg
  iron, copper, zinc, selenium, chromium, boron, manganese, iodine and potassium

Drugs Can Deplete Nutrients

Today, more than ever before, Americans are gulping down drugs (prescription and nonprescription, or over-the-counter) in record amounts. All one has to do is watch television one night. Headaches, runny noses, sore throats, constipation, diarrhea, upset stomach, allergies and sinus problems, etc., can all be overcome by downing Drug A or Drug B, on down to Drug Z.

What America does not realize is that many of these drugs actually cause depletion of the body's essential vitamins and minerals. A recent scientific study shows that ingredients found in common over-the-counter (OTC) cold, pain and allergy remedies actually lower the blood level of vitamin A in animals. Because vitamin A protects and strengthens the mucous membranes lining the nose, throat and lungs, a deficiency of vitamin A could actually break down these membranes, giving bacteria a cozy home to multiply in. Therefore, the drugs that are supposed to alleviate the cold may be actually prolonging it!

Side effects of drugs are well known. Antihistamines can cause drowsiness; aspirin can cause stomach upset.

But what most of us do not know is that they can also cause a nutritional deficiency. Many drugs either stop the absorption of nutrients or interfere with the cells' ability to use them.

Which Drugs Deplete Vitamins and Minerals?

ASPIRIN

Millions of pounds of aspirin are consumed every year in America. It is a common ingredient in many prescription and nonprescription pain relievers, cold remedies, and sinus remedies. A study has shown that even a small amount of aspirin can *triple* the excretion rate of vitamin C from the body.

Many millions take aspirin to relieve the pain and inflammation of arthritis. What they don't know is that aspirin not only depletes the body of vitamin C, but can also lead to a deficiency of folic acid, one of the B vitamins. A deficiency of folic acid can lead to anemia, digestive disturbances, graying hair and even growth problems.

CORTICOSTEROIDS

Corticosteroids such as cortisone and prednisone belong to another class of drugs used to ease the pain of arthritis. They are also prescribed for skin problems, blood and eye disorders and asthma. Researchers conducted a study of 24 asthmatics using cortisone-type drugs and found the zinc levels were 42 percent lower than in patients not treated with corticosteroids.

A zinc deficiency can lead to loss of taste and smell as well as a loss of sexual desire. Zinc is necessary for male potency and the health of the prostate gland. Zinc also enhances wound healing and is essential for a clear complexion.

THE PILL

These oral contraceptives are made from a synthetic hormone that can lead to a deficiency of zinc, folic acid and vitamins C, B6 and B12. Deficiency of B12 can lead to a nervous condition. B6 deficiency can cause depression—many women on the pill are depressed. Women taking oral contraceptives (birth control pills) should take at least 25–30 mg of B6, 4 mg of B12, 800 mg of folic acid and 1,000 mg of vitamin C. Low vitamin C levels may account for increased susceptibility to blood clotting.

BARBITURATES (PHENOBARB, SECONAL, NEMBUTAL, BUTISOL)

These are strong sedatives and hypnotics which are prescribed for insomnia. A study done reveals that a significant number of people tested who took barbiturates had low calcium levels. A lack of calcium can cause osteoporosis and muscle cramps.

LAXATIVES AND ANTACIDS

These are routinely prescribed for digestive complaints, constipation or ulcers. Antacids that contain aluminum disturb calcium and phosphorus metabolism. Phosphorus deficiency, which is very rare (except in antacid users), can cause fatigue, loss of appetite and fragile bones.

MINERAL OIL (a LUBRICANT LAXATIVE)

Mineral oil used as a laxative prevents absorption of vitamins A and D. Any laxative taken to excess can flush out large amounts of potassium, which can cause heart problems and muscle weakness.

DIURETICS

Diuretics, which are commonly prescribed for high blood pressure, also flush potassium out of the body. And antibiotics can also rob the body of potassium.

THE TEN MOST COMMON SIDE EFFECTS OF PRESCRIPTION DRUGS

The following are the most frequently reported side effects of the top 100 pharmaceutical drugs. If you have any of these symptoms, ask your M.D. if they could be caused by the drugs you are taking.

1. Skin rash
2. Nausea/vomiting
3. Diarrhea
4. Dizziness
5. Stomach pain, cramps
6. Headache
7. Insomnia
8. Constipation
9. Hypotension (low blood pressure)
10. Drowsiness
11. Itching

Newer Nutrients

The field of nutrition is experiencing an amazing information explosion, with our knowledge *doubling* about every eighteen months. Exciting research discoveries are made almost daily—here is some of the good news about vitamins and minerals:

- More than 90 studies have now linked vitamins with a reduced cancer risk. One 35-year study of 2,000 men showed a sevenfold protective effect for beta carotene.
- A University of California study found that vitamin C prevents sperm damage that causes sterility
- *The New England Journal of Medicine* reported that calcium supplementation significantly slowed the weakening of bones from osteoporosis
- Johns Hopkins researchers found that vitamin E halves the risk of developing cataracts

Here are some of the nutrients whose value has been discovered in recent years.

Inosine

♦ Heightens ATP, which elevates your energy level while it helps delay muscle fatigue

Di- and Tri-methyl Glycine

♦ Increases peak performance by increasing oxygen transportation
♦ Can delay lactic acid buildup which causes muscle fatigue
♦ Tri-methyl is more active than di-methylglycine

Chondroitin Sulfate (CSA), A Mucopolysaccharide

♦ Important for rehabilitation of the musculoskeletal system
♦ Aids the cardiovascular system

Coenzyme Q10

♦ Reduces the risk of heart attack
♦ Stimulates the immune system
♦ Aids in the treatment of periodontal disease
♦ Lowers blood pressure
♦ Antioxidant similar to vitamin E
♦ Aids in the prevention of toxicity from drugs used to treat aging

Cytochrome-C

♦ A carrier of oxygen
♦ Increases the length of time muscles will not fatigue

Dibencozide

♦ A precursor of vitamin B12; can be well absorbed if taken by mouth

Octocosanol

♦ Active ingredient of wheat germ
♦ Important for physical stamina

Pyridoxal-5 Phosphate

♦ Coenzyme form of pyridoxine (B6)
♦ It is the most usable form of B6

Yohimbine

♦ The only known aphrodisiac for men
♦ Seems to have the ability to improve production of testosterone, the male sex hormone
♦ Yohimbine is available by prescription—but only in the USA
♦ Yohimbine bark is available without a prescription

Vitamin and Mineral Thieves

The following is a list of drugs that induce *vitamin and mineral deficiencies* and the nutrients they deplete. Look it over before you take your next medicine.

THIEVING DRUG	NUTRIENTS DEPLETED
Alcohol (including alcohol-containing cough syrups, elixirs, and OTC medications such as Nyquil)	Vitamins A, B1, B2, biotin, choline, niacin, vitamin B15, folic acid, & magnesium
Ammonium Chloride (e.g., Ambenyl, Expectorant, Triaminicol, decongestant cough syrup, P.V. Tussin Syrup)	Vitamin C
Antacids (e.g., Maalox, Mylanta, Gelusil, Tums, Rolaids)	B complex, vitamin A
Anticoagulants (e.g., Coumadin, Dicumarol, Panwarfin)	Vitamins A, K
Antihistamines (e.g., Chlor-Trimeton, Pyribenzamine)	Vitamin C

Aspirin (and remember, APC drugs contain aspirin)	Vitamins A, B complex, C, calcium, potassium
Barbiturates (e.g., Phenobarbital, Seconal, Nembutal, Butisol)	Vitamins A, C, D, folic acid
Caffeine (present in all APC medicines)	Vitamin B1, inositol, biotin, potassium, zinc; can also inhibit calcium and iron assimilation; vitamin K, niacin
Chloramphenicol (Chlomycetin)	
Cholestyramine (Questran)	Vitamins A, D, E, K, potassium
Cimetidine (Tagamet)	Vitamin B1
Clofibrate (Atromid-S)	Vitamin K
Colchicine (Colbenemid)	B12, A, potassium
Diethylstilbestrol (DES)	Vitamin B6
Diuretics (e.g., Diuril, Hydrodiuril, Ser-Ap-Es, Lasix)	B complex, potassium, magnesium, zinc
Fluorides	Vitamin C
Glutethimide (Doriden)	Folic acid
Indomethacin (Indocin)	Vitamins B1 and C
Isoniazid (INH, Nydrazind)	Vitamin B6
Kanamycin (Kantrex)	Vitamins K, B12
Laxatives, lubricants (e.g., castor oil mineral oil)	Vitamins A, D, E, K, calcium, phosphorus
Meprednisone (Betapar)	Vitamins B6, C, zinc, potassium

Methotrexate (Mexate)	Folic acid
Nitrofurantoin (e.g., Furadantin, Macrodantin)	Folic acid
Oral contraceptives (e.g., Brevicon, Demulen, Enovid, Lo/ovral, Norinyl, Ovral)	Folic acid, vitamins C, B2, B6, B12, E
Penicillamine (Cuprimine)	Vitamin B6
Penicillin (in all its forms)	Vitamins B6, K, niacin
Phenylbutazone (e.g., Azolid, Butazolidin)	Folic acid
Phenytoin (Dilantin)	Folic acid, vitamin D
Prednisone (e.g., Meticorten, Prednisolone, Orasone)	Vitamins B6, D, C, zinc, potassium
Propantheline (Pro-Banthine)	Vitamin K
Pyrimethamine (Daraprim)	Folic acid
Sulfonamides, systemic (e.g., Bactrim, Gantanol, Tantrisin, Septra)	Folic acid, vitamins K, B2
Sulfonamides and topical steroids (e.g., Aerosporin, Cortisporin, Neosporin, Polysporin)	Vitamins K, B12, folic acid
Tetracyclines (e.g., Achromycin-V, Sumycin, Tetracyn)	Vitamin K, calcium, magnesium, iron
Tobacco	Vitamins C, B1, folic acid, calcium
Trifluoperazine (Stelazine)	Vitamin B12
Triamterene (Dyrenium)	Folic acid

INDEX

116